Pure Romance
Between the Sheets

Disclaimer

All names have been changed (except where noted) to protect the privacy of those referred to in this book. In addition, all individuals and couples are referred to in heterosexual terms, but the author and Pure Romance respect and include people of all sexual orientations in the creation and production of their products, as well as the advice included in this book.

Pure Romance Between the Sheets

Find Your Best Sexual Self and Enhance Your Intimate Relationship

PATTY BRISBEN

ATRIA PAPERBACK

New York   London   Toronto   Sydney

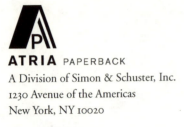

ATRIA PAPERBACK

A Division of Simon & Schuster, Inc.
1230 Avenue of the Americas
New York, NY 10020

First Atria Paperback edition June 2010

ATRIA PAPERBACK and colophon are trademarks of Simon & Schuster, Inc.

For information about special discounts for bulk purchases,
please contact Simon & Schuster Special Sales at
1-866-506-1949 or business@simonandschuster.com.

The Simon & Schuster Speakers Bureau can bring authors to your live event. For
more information or to book an event contact the Simon & Schuster Speakers
Bureau at 1-866-248-3049 or visit our website at www.simonspeakers.com.

Designed by Davina Mock-Maniscalco

Manufactured in the United States of America

10 9 8 7 6 5 4 3 2 1

The Library of Congress has cataloged the hardcover edition as follows:

Brisben, Patty.
    Pure romance between the sheets : find your best sexual self and enhance your
intimate relationship / by Patty Brisben.—1st ed.
        p.   cm.
    Includes bibliographical references.
    1. Women.   2. Sex.   3. Sexual attraction.   4. Identity (Psychology).
I. Title.

HQ1155.B75   2008
613.9'6082—dc22   2008014122

ISBN 978-1-4165-7263-3 (pbk)

This book is dedicated to those who have devoted their lives and careers to helping women have a happier, healthier understanding of their bodies, intimate relationships, and sexual health. Their passion and commitment have paved the way for all to embrace their sexuality with confidence, clarity, and courage.

Contents

PART TWO

Turning to Your Relationship

Pure Romance
Between the Sheets

Introduction

ON 1983 I was on maternity leave from my job at a pediatrician's office, home one day with my four kids. I was an average middle-class housewife, happy and busy enough. My three boys were outside playing in the backyard, and my new baby daughter was napping inside the house with me when I happened to flip on the TV. Phil Donahue was interviewing a couple of women about their new, sideline careers, which were making a huge difference in their lives. They spoke about how empowering it was to sell their products to women and how these items seemed to be boosting women's self-esteem and strengthening their relationships.

As I paid more attention, I began to understand that these very normal looking ladies were throwing Tupperware-style parties for their friends, where they would present an array of items that women and men could use to enhance sexual pleasure—they were selling lubricants, vibrators, and other toys!

I couldn't believe my ears. And aside from the provocative subject matter, what really got my attention was how confident and self-assured these women sounded.

Later that day, I called my friend Nancy to find out what time our sons' Little League game was. After exchanging logistical info for the baseball game, I said, "Hey, Nancy, did you happen to see Phil Donahue? Do you know who he had on today?"

Nancy had not caught the show. "Can you believe it," I asked. "I mean, who in her right mind would use any of those things?" As I rambled on, I was becoming increasingly uncomfortable by Nancy's silence—I thought I had offended her.

Finally my friend said, "Actually, Patty, I went to one of those parties just the other night in Old Milford."

I was shocked for two reasons—first that my friend had actually gone to such a party and second that such a party had taken place in a small Ohio town.

"Were there a lot of people at the party?" I asked.

"It was packed," she said.

"But no one bought anything, right?"

"Well, actually, the line went out the door!" Nancy said.

You could have knocked me over with a feather.

"But *you* didn't buy anything, did you?" I expected her to say, "Oh, nothing. You know me."

Instead she said, "I bought a vibrator."

After exchanging a few more pleasantries, we hung up, leaving me a bit flabbergasted. "If Nancy could buy a vibrator . . ."

So began my crash course in the land of bedroom toys. I had asked Nancy for the company's contact information, and somewhat nervously, I called the company and ordered a Starter Kit for becoming a sales consultant, just to see what was included. After I hung up, I was still anxious. How was I going to cover the cost of these products? It wasn't like we had money to spare from our family budget, especially since I was on maternity leave. But then

I thought about the women I'd seen on Phil Donahue. Maybe I could become a part of a business that not only helped women but made money too! So I picked up the phone again and began calling all my friends to invite them to a party. I scheduled it for one week after the date I was supposed to receive my starter kit.

When my husband came home from work that night, I told him all about the show and how I was going to make lots of money with this new business. He looked at me like I was crazy and said, "No wife of mine is going to do this sort of thing. You must still have the baby blues or something. You better cancel that order."

I tried to explain that I really wanted to give this a try—not to mention that it was a perfect solution to finding more quality time with my kids *and* making money. "And besides," I said, "I made a commitment and I'm going to do this."

Despite my husband's lack of support, I was determined to go through with my plan.

But once my products arrived, I got nervous all over again. What if no one showed up at the party? How was I going to justify all the money I'd spent? So again, I picked up the phone and called more women I knew in the community, coming up with a total of twenty women. By the night of the party, twenty had turned into forty! The house was packed and everyone had a blast. And I knew I was onto something—something very special indeed.

That was over twenty-five years ago. My husband and I went our separate ways, and like many women today, I became a woman who wears at least three hats—as a mother, businesswoman, and sex educator. As a mother, I have raised four children to be knowledgeable, confident, and respectful of their sexuality. As a businesswoman, I founded Pure Romance, Inc., creating hundreds of sex-enhancing products that respond to women's and men's needs, netting over $80 million in sales. And finally, as a sex educator, I have spent twenty-five years listening to women and answering their questions about sex. Through my network of party consultants and our dynamic website (www.pureromance.com), I have created a safe, trustworthy place for women of all ages and from all walks of life to air their fears, disclose confusion, and find reliable, accurate information that has the power to transform their lives.

I am both proud and humbled by all this success. And though the phenomenal growth of my company has been quite a rollercoaster ride for a single mom of four, it's the ever-growing family of women whom I have encountered and truly want to reach that really mean the most to me. What began as a simple party is now a mission to educate, empower, and inspire women to respect and treasure one of the most vital aspects of their lives: their sexuality.

When I started selling relationship enhancement products, I read every single book I could find about women, their bodies, and relationships. The more time I spent on the road, listening and talking to women, hearing their stories, and answering their questions, the more clearly I saw that there was a gap between buying these enhancement products and truly knowing what to do with them. In other words, most of the women I was meeting in this early part of my career didn't just want to purchase a bedroom toy to add a bit of spice to their love life, they needed to know how to use that toy, how to introduce it into their relationship without feeling awkward or afraid, and perhaps most important, how to feel comfortable in their own skin when it came to their sexuality. I soon realized that for all the people selling products and writing books on sex tips, there was no good source for women to reach out to to make sense of this information in a personal way. Tips, techniques, and products can make a great evening of sex, but if a woman can't also connect to an inner place where her sexuality makes sense to her, then all that information has the power of simply a good, one-night stand.

Consider these two statistics:

♡ A survey of 125 U.S. and sixteen Canadian medical schools revealed that the majority of undergraduate medical programs provide less than ten hours of education on human sexuality. This explains the challenge many women encounter when they pose specific sex-related questions to their doctors: their doctors don't know enough about sex!

♡ A survey of adults twenty-five years of age and above showed that 85 percent would like to discuss a sexual problem with their physician, but 68 percent were reluctant to ask and 71 percent thought their concerns would be dismissed. Talk about a trust problem and a communication gap!

I am here to fill that gap. Women turn to me because they trust me and feel comfortable sharing their most personal and intimate issues. They continue to come back because they know they can access accurate information that makes sense and works in their lives. My consultants and I are out in the field talking and listening to thousands of women. We hear what women want firsthand and so we have become their go-to source for information about anything sexual. They may be embarrassed to ask their friends, or afraid of getting unreliable or inaccurate information, and they may even shy away from discussing such things with their partners. And we know many are not turning to their doctors! Again, what I've realized over the past twenty-five years in the field is that what these thousands of women logging onto our website and attending our parties are really asking for is trustworthy, accurate information that makes sense to *them*. So when I founded my own company, I made certain that every single one of the consultants who sold my products was rigorously trained. I sought out the best and brightest experts, and developed a systematic training code and program so that when one of my 20,000 plus consultants hosts a party, leads a workshop, or presents to a lecture hall of college students, they offer not only techniques and products for sexual enhancement, but also a way for women to understand the very nature of their sexuality.

All that Pure Romance has brought to me has made me want to give back to the community at large. With that in mind, I have established two outreach programs and a not-for-profit organization within Pure Romance, each focused on sexual health issues for a specific audience. The Patty Brisben Foundation contributes funds to various charitable causes and supports ongoing breast cancer and sexual health research; Sensuality, Sexuality, Survival was designed for women following cancer diagnosis and treatment; and The Naked Truth is part of a national college tour presentation aimed at delivering sexual health information to college students on their campuses—as I like to say, "get the truth before you get naked!" And through collaborative research studies with Indiana University (home of the Kinsey Institute), Pure Romance has helped hundreds of thousands of women live fuller, healthier, more satisfying lives.

To me, sexuality is one of the foundations of a woman's sense of her own power, and when we truly learn to own, honor, and respect this vital aspect of ourselves, we enrich every aspect and dimension of our lives. Yes, tips, toys, and techniques can lead us to great sexual pleasure, but that pleasure will not last unless it comes with an inner foundation of awareness and knowledge.

Educating and empowering women has always been the mission and promise of my company, and now I want to share all that with you in this book. I want *Pure Romance* to be a road map for your own "inner journey," so that you too can develop the self-knowledge, the confidence, and the wisdom to make your sexuality a fulfilling part of your life, for the rest of your life.

When you make this shift, and learn how to embrace the inner foundation of your sexuality, you empower your relationship with your partner; you increase your confidence to achieve your personal and professional goals; and you enrich your sense of self. So many women have come to me and said, "Thank you!" Not because they had a great night of intimacy with their partner, but because they rediscovered themselves and found a new way to live to their fullest potential. And that is the heart and soul of my promise. After taking care of my kids, I have completely devoted myself to helping women believe in themselves and find the pleasure and power that come from truly owning their sexuality. And this requires not just learning the ins and outs of lubricants, vibrators, and other bedroom toys (all of which you will soon find out), but really understanding your sexuality during all the stages of your life.

Part One, This Is for You, focuses on helping you understand your own sexuality and how your body works. I will show you how to get in touch with how you like to be touched, how to think about your libido or desire, and even how best to trigger your arousal and reach orgasm. As you understand more about how orgasms happen, you will learn how to increase your orgasmic pleasure. And if you've never had an orgasm, you may just find what's been in the way. Most important, you will know how to think about orgasms—so you can keep the "almighty O" in perspective.

In four succinct chapters, women will get much closer to understanding what's going on with their bodies and their minds when it comes to sex:

Getting in Your Comfort Zone About Sex

Your Love, Your Life, Your Libido

Beyond the Bedroom: Taking Responsibility for Your
   Sexual Health

Putting the "O" Back in Romance

In Part Two, Turning to Your Relationship, I expand the discussion about sex to be more of an intimacy guide for women who are now ready to apply their self-knowledge to their relationship. If you're not in a relationship right now, you may still find these chapters useful as a way to help hone what you want in a future relationship. These five chapters will help prepare you to be your best sexual self with someone you trust and care about:

Pillow Talk: Learning How to Stay Close

"Your Body Is a Wonderland": Discovering the Power
   of Touch

Pure Pleasure: Lubrication Education

Batteries Not Included: The World of Toys

Moving Beyond Missionary: Expanding Your Pleasure

You'll have all the information you need to know how to make your intimate relationship the fun, trusting, loving place it should be.

Again, though some of the topics may seem familiar, especially those in Part Two, what's new and absolutely different from any sex book out there is the lens through which I deliver the information. After reading this book, you will walk away not with a list of tips in your head, but with a complete understanding of your sexuality and how you want to use these tips. You will walk away with the confidence and trust in yourself that before you have only dreamt about.

Everything you will learn in these pages is based on solid, medically sound research and findings from our own research sources, combined with what we access through our affiliations with Indiana University (home of the Kinsey Institute) and the American Association of Sexual Educators, Counselors, and Therapists (AASECT). In addition, within each chapter, I highlight the most commonly asked questions selected from my "Ask Patty" column on the Pure Romance website. These questions cover a range of topics, including some basic "how-to" questions regarding how to introduce bedroom toys or how to have a clitoral orgasm. Some are more medically oriented questions such as how to overcome pain during sex and what birth control is suitable for someone on antidepressants. Other questions are more relationship oriented and will help you solve intimacy issues that might be surfacing with your partner.

I have also included "Intimacy Issues." Based on my twenty-five years in the field, these "issues" are common hang-ups that often get in the way of women fully experiencing and enjoying their sexuality. Some are related to emotional issues, others are medical or health-related questions.

Pure Romance is my gift to all you out there who want to learn not only how to achieve sexual pleasure, but how and why this knowledge can help you understand your body, your mind, and that wonderful, sometimes confusing relationship between the two.

PART ONE

This Is For You

CHAPTER ONE

Under the Covers

Getting into Your Comfort Zone about Sex

OR YEARS NOW, I have been keeping women's sexual secrets. They trust me with their questions, their fears, and their stories—and I take this trust to heart. I understand that talking about sex can make some women feel uncomfortable, but it doesn't have to. In fact, if we take the subject from behind closed doors and treat it with the respect and the care it deserves, we will do ourselves a big favor. We will also get much closer to one of my goals: to make sex—and talking about sex—a natural part of the web of life—something completely normal, special, and fun!

Why do most women trust me when it comes to anything sexual? For two reasons: First, for more than two decades, I've been on the front lines, working with women (initially as a sales consultant and later as the founder of Pure Romance) to provide advice on safe sexual practices and how to become more intimate with their partners. Second, in my newer role as a national speaker, I make a point of speaking about sex as if I were talking about any other subject—the weather, the perfect pair of high heels, or my dream vacation. I believe that by making sex an approachable, natural subject worthy of a conversation, I can show women how much they can gain from becoming more comfortable around the topic. I want them—and you—to know that the more you learn about your own body and how you respond to stimulation; the more you understand how lubricants can relieve dryness and enhance pleasure; the more you see how introducing a simple bedroom accessory can lead you to experience deeper sensation, more pleasure, or your first orgasm; and the more you gain insight into how to reconnect with your partner so you can enjoy one another again—the more you will feel grounded, satisfied, and fulfilled in your life.

It's our right as women to own our sexuality—and it's also our responsibility. Our sexuality has the power to be an intense source of pleasure throughout our lives. How can I be so sure of this? Because after twenty-five years of sharing sexual information with women, I have seen thousands transformed by this knowledge. I've watched hundreds of women leave a Pure Romance party, saying, "I didn't know it was going to be like this" or "I didn't know I was missing so much" or "I didn't know sex could be so easy and so fun!" Surprise, elation, and determination ring in their voices. And that's what keeps me going. That, and wanting to reach more and more women.

This book offers something for every one of you. If you are seeking information about how to become aroused, what to do if you frequently feel dry or irritated, or how to subtly introduce a lubricant or bedroom toy—you will find both the know-how and the insight in these pages. And whatever situation you're in right now—newly married or newly divorced, recently widowed or still single, just given birth or facing an illness or surgery—you will discover the secret to your comfort zone so that you can become the confident, caring lover you always knew you could be.

I am making only one request: that you consider the significance and the importance of your sexuality in terms of who *you* are. Don't compare yourself to your friends, your sisters, your mother, or your daughter. Simply get to know your body, your mind, your sexuality. My challenge to you is this: Would you rather embrace this powerful dimension of what makes you a woman and let it lead you to a wonderful, full life or let it stay hidden and untapped, weighing you down in body and spirit?

In the pages that follow, I want you to open yourself to the possibility of embarking on this fun, fantastic adventure, one in which you will get to know yourself better—physically, emotionally, and sexually. Yes, you will learn some great tips and techniques that can resuscitate a relationship that's lost its spark and drive you and your partner wild, but more than that, you will come away with greater insight and confidence in your sexuality and the central place it should have in your life.

How Do You Think About Sex?

For many women, even bringing up the subject of sex makes them shut down. Most of the time this is related to their background and how they first learned—or didn't learn—about sex. Women who were raised in an environment where sex was taboo or treated as shameful often have a hard time letting go of those negative feelings. This may sound obvious, but I can't tell you how many women treat their sexuality as a negative thing, hiding from it themselves or keeping it hidden from others. They are blocked from truly embracing their sexuality because they judge it as something bad, dirty, or morally wrong. As Pam, a forty-two-year-old mother of two, said to me, "My parents never mentioned the word 'sex,' and I was just too afraid to ask any questions. I just assumed sex was a topic you weren't supposed to talk about."

When I visited Indiana University on my first college tour, I had a remarkable experience with a woman who wasn't aware that she actually had negative associations with sex. Dr. Michael Reece, a professor and director of the Center for Sexual Health Promotion at Indiana University, and part of our research team at Pure Romance, had assembled over four hundred students for my presentation. Before the seminar, the students had been asked to complete a rather explicit survey about their sexual interests and behaviors. They were asked such questions as: "Have you ever gone into an adult bookstore? If so, did you purchase any adult toys? Have you used one with yourself? Have you ever shopped online? Have you ever had an orgasm?"

Before introducing me to the assembled students, Dr. Reece delivered some of the results from the survey: "Seventy-eight percent of you said you shopped online or had been to an adult store; 32 percent bought a bedroom toy, etc." Then Dr. Reece asked whether the audience was interested in learning more about sex and toys. Everyone gave a resounding "Yes!" (I'm sure they also knew the founder of Pure Romance was about to take the stage!) Next, he said, "I have one final question. Do you think learning about sex and thinking about buying bedroom toys contributes to society?"

One woman raised her hand immediately and said, "I don't think there is any reason for sex toys of any kind. They simply demoralize women and there is no need for such products."

A bit of silence followed and then I walked to the podium. I began as I often do by asking how many of them ever took medicine when they get a cold or the flu. Most hands shot up. I then asked if they were aware that over-the-counter antihistamines not only closed and dried up their nasal passages but also the lubrication that is natural to their other orifices (i.e., the sex organs!). Most people just shook their heads. Next, I asked how many of them often felt stressed before an exam, returning home after a semester away, or even managing the balance between a job and school. Most hands again shot up. "Did you know that any kind of stress can also make your body dry and make it difficult for you to respond sexually? And that by introducing a lubricant, you can immediately and profoundly change the experience of sex?" Heads began nodding in understanding. Finally I asked, "And how many of you would like to know more about finding your partner's hot spot of pleasure? Would you like to know more about what turns you on and gets you aroused? Did you know that by introducing certain bedroom accessories you can find out this information quickly and easily? Have you ever wondered why there are hundreds of varieties of shampoo and conditioners? Because we are all different—with different likes and dislikes, different needs and desires. The same rule applies to lubricants and bedroom accessories."

At the end of my presentation, while I was lingering at the front of the enormous room, I looked up and saw the woman who had first raised her hand barreling down the aisle. I admit, I was actually a bit scared. Dr. Reece moved closer to me as if to protect me. But when she was close enough for me to see her face, I knew what had happened. She grabbed my hand and said, "Thank you so much! You have changed my mind. I didn't know I was so uncomfortable about sex—I thought I had it all together. Before, I thought lubricants and sex toys were for 'other' kinds of women. But the way you describe them, I see now how incredibly helpful—and enjoyable—they can be. I didn't realize I had so much to learn. I feel like my world has opened up."

Dr. Reece turned to me and said, "I can offer a ton of information, but I can't change a person's point of view like you just did."

In one two-hour presentation, this woman had accomplished a major shift in her thinking. Instead of judging the subject matter of the talk (and probably the speaker as well!) and rejecting the possibility that she might actually enjoy herself, she succeeded in opening her mind to learning about herself and what she wanted. In place of negative thoughts and a closed mind, she now had a desire to explore. And that's what I want to instill in you.

Not every one of you will want to run out and get a vibrator (though by the end of this book, you might just be persuaded!) or learn how to resuscitate your relationship in twenty-four hours, but if you simply open your mind and your heart to the possibility that you don't already know everything about your sexuality, then you will be giving yourself a remarkable gift: the gift of learning something new about yourself that can lead to a richer, fuller, more meaningful life.

Eyes Wide Open

Although I adjust my presentations according to who is in my audience—whether that be college-age women (and men), women in their thirties, forties, and fifties who are juggling marriage, careers, and kids, or whether I am talking to a vulnerable yet proud group of cancer survivors, my goal is always the same: to help them become aware that there is a lot that they can do to make their sexual experience both more fulfilling and more pleasurable. And that the more they know about what can change and what they can add to their experience, the more in control and empowered they will feel.

That is what learning about sex can do for you, too. It can open all the doors of your life. And this is as true for young, college-age women as it is for more mature women. Like Mariam, a thirty-something mother of a pair of twins, who approached me after a Pure Romance party. I had watched her throughout the evening, and although she had smiled and laughed with the rest of the group, she also hung back, appearing reluctant to jump into the party spirit. Near the end of the evening, I wasn't surprised to find her standing by my side.

"Patty," Mariam said quietly, "I've been married almost ten years and my relationship with my husband has gotten really bad. He thinks I'm frigid." And she began to cry.

I quickly consoled her, saying, "First off, I doubt that's the case if you're here tonight. Why don't you tell me what's been going on?"

It turns out that after her two sons were born, Mariam had started to feel more and more uncomfortable about sex. It was almost as if she felt bad when she was being sexual, that it would somehow make her a bad mother. At first, her husband was sympathetic and gave her lots of room, thinking it was just a "phase." But almost six years later, he had lost his patience and his feelings of sympathy had turned to anger and frustration.

"He knows I came here tonight, but I think he's given up hope. I'm afraid he's going to leave me."

Mariam's situation is much more common than you might think. Here was a woman in her physical prime, with some un-

derstanding of how things had veered off track in her sexual relationship, but she didn't know how to set things right. I could tell
that she and her husband had not fallen out of love, but rather
that she had lost touch with herself. I asked Mariam if she thought
of herself as a sexual person and her response was "sort of." I understood that to mean, "I don't know what it is to be a sexual
person." I then asked her a few more questions about her background and discovered, not surprisingly, that she had been raised
in a fairly conservative household. "We never talked about sex.
And my parents didn't seem close—they were never affectionate
with each other," Mariam explained.

When I asked her how sexuality fit into her life, she said quietly, "I just don't think about it very much."

"Would you like to be more sexual?" I knew I was going out
on a limb, but I felt it was very important for Mariam to recognize
that though she came from a family that had a negative, judgmental view of sexuality and may not have been loving in a physical
way, she had a choice—a choice to have a different relationship
with her husband.

"Yes, I would," she said, smiling a bit nervously.

When I saw that smile—and I get a lot of smiles—I knew
that she had begun her own journey of truly owning her sexuality.
Sometimes all we need is a gentle push to open up and share our
story or our feelings or experiences. But that first step is essential.
I admired the courage it took Mariam to say "Yes" and I admired
the confidence she was beginning to build. Before we went our
separate ways, I offered Mariam some suggestions for how to learn
more about herself sexually (you'll learn more about this later in
the chapter), and then I drove home my main point: You've got to
give yourself permission to be sexual. Nothing could be healthier

for your family than your children knowing that their parents are truly and joyously connected—in every way.

Let me share another story about how, no matter how deeply rooted one's negative attitude toward sex may be, there is still the possibility to change. Lynette (her real name) was a fifty-something woman from Wisconsin who for twenty-five years had been active in her church, even serving as the leader of its choir. For a quarter of a century, her entire life had revolved around the church. As she said, "My life has been about serving wherever I can." But after suffering through a brain tumor and also watching a dear friend struggle unsuccessfully against breast cancer, Lynette risked her ties to her church because of how deeply moved she was by her new mission to serve as a Pure Romance consultant. As she described so boldly in a letter to us, she could not help her friend, "But it wasn't too late for me." After being introduced to a Pure Romance consultant, she realized "I was too embarrassed to talk about sex to anyone, even my doctor. I just wasn't comfortable discussing that area of my life. . . . But I was so impressed by the consultant's compassion toward women, I found myself telling her things that I never discussed with anyone else. She immediately suggested that I try one of the bedroom accessories, and I did and it changed my life. It was as if I finally gave myself permission to think of myself as a sexual person."

Lynette became a Pure Romance consultant because, as she said, "I felt given what both my girlfriend and I went through, then there must be loads of people who are looking for the information that can help them." And when Lynette was asked to leave her church and give up her role as choir leader, she said this: "My dedication to service kicked in again, and I believed that I could do a job that was actually helping people. . . . My focus is to educate women with information they seek, . . . and when people tell me how [I have helped] them strengthen their marriage, that is the greatest reward."

Obviously you don't have to become a Pure Romance consultant to benefit from the information in this book; nor do you have to buy a single product. All you need to do is embrace the power and wisdom the women in these pages have to offer you.

Intimacy Issue #1—"Don't Touch Yourself."

Many of us have heard this refrain from our mothers, fathers, or siblings, or we say it to ourselves. It's time to banish those chastising voices in your head once and for all! Remember Lynette's story? It's never too early—or too late—to give yourself permission to explore your body and understand your sexuality more fully.

Clare is a perfect example of a woman who is so distant from her sexuality that she had never felt lust or sexual desire—never mind turned on enough to experience an orgasm. Working with her Pure Romance consultant, she slowly but surely opened the door of her sexuality and found a passionate, eager woman inside. But this process took a while. As Clare said, "I had never ever touched myself. I was brought up to believe that it was just plain wrong. So when I got married, I had no idea what I liked. I just assumed sex was something I did for my husband. It was my duty as a wife. But when a friend of mine invited me to a Pure Romance party, I went along—really just to be a good friend. At first, when the women started discussing vibrators and other bedroom accessories, I thought they were crazy. I felt so uncomfortable I wanted to run out of the room. But other women at the party were sharing their stories of how much their lives—and their relationships—had changed. So I bought a small vibrator and tried using it that afternoon—when my husband was still at work and the kids were not yet home from school. I know this sounds completely unbelievable, but I had never felt so great. I think my first orgasm was a complete accident! I have never felt so excited in my life, and learning to be more open in this way has literally changed my marriage."

Getting in touch with your sexuality is not as simple as turning on a faucet. It's about making a commitment to explore yourself, your desires, and how you respond to stimulation—in all ways. It can take time, but it's a process that can lead you to enormous pleasure. As you will see in the next chapter, one of the first steps to learning more about yourself is masturbation.

Your Comfort Zone

When women give themselves permission to be sexual, they have the key to finding and defining their comfort zone. So whether you are a woman whose challenge is getting back in touch with yourself after childbirth or you've never fully understood or appreciated the role of sexuality in your life, you can learn to give yourself permission to value and honor this important part of who you are. If you are in your twenties, then you have your whole life ahead of you! Do you know how many women would have killed for this information when they were twenty-five?! As

Gwynne, twenty-eight, said, "I am so much more confident knowing what my choices are."

In order to find your comfort zone about sex, you must give yourself permission to learn—about yourself, first of all. And what do I mean exactly by finding your comfort zone? I mean feeling at ease with your sexual needs and desires; being comfortable in your own skin; comfortable talking about your sexuality with your partner or best friend; comfortable asking a new partner to use protection and practice safe sex; and comfortable finding out how to take care of your sexual health.

Some women operate outside their comfort zone because they simply never learned enough about sex and were taught that "good" girls should not be curious about it. Others married young and quickly had children, and they never bothered or found the time to investigate this side of themselves. I want you to come to the realization that curiosity is healthy and necessary—it's not only a goal but also an attitude that will uncover so many wonderful things during the course of your life.

Let Me Introduce You to Your Sexual Self

Like many things that make us grow, there is a process involved in truly understanding your sexuality. And you need to be clear on where you've been to know where you want to go. So as you begin to think about who you are, sexually speaking, consider these questions:

1. When was your first sexual experience?

2. Was it positive or negative? Pleasurable or painful?

3. Where or from whom did you learn about sex?

4. Did you experiment with self stimulation?

5. Have you ever experienced sex without your consent?

6. Do you ever experience pain with sex?

7. Do you like sex or do you go "go through the motions"?

8. Have you ever had a completely wonderful experience during sex?

9. Have you ever had an orgasm?

10. If you are in a relationship, do you feel that your partner understands you sexually?

There are no right or wrong answers to these questions. There are simply your answers. By answering these questions, you are focusing your attention on your own sexual experience. And when was the last time you gave it any thought? Most of us spend our days running around, balancing work with taking care of kids or partners, pets, elderly parents, or all of the above. Once the day is done, dinner's over, and the kitchen cleaned up, the last thing on our minds is sex! Who has the time or the energy?

I always tell women this: If you're going to participate in sex, you should enjoy it. So this book is not about overthinking your sexuality; it's about making it simple—and making it better. Use the questions above as a guide to helping you discern where you've been in terms of your sexuality and where you are now. Then, slowly but surely, open that door to new ways to think about your sexuality.

The truth of the matter is that if we spend some quiet time just with ourselves and begin to become more aware of our sexuality, we will be more in control of how we approach our sexuality. We can learn to make vital decisions about what we want and what we need. For instance, if your response to the first question was, "I first had sex when I was seventeen," and you are now in your mid-thirties, do you know that your body has changed dramatically over the intervening fifteen-plus years? If you answered the second question by saying that your first sexual encounter was "pleasurable," then good for you! For many women, the first sexual experience tends to be not only frightening but also painful. These early experiences can have a profound impact on how we think about sex. As one woman told me, "I first had sex when I was sixteen. My boyfriend kept pressuring me and pressuring me, so I finally gave in. I didn't really know what I was doing, but looking back, I think having sex so early made it difficult for me to trust men. I always thought about sex as something *they* wanted—it had nothing to do with me. It wasn't until I married and my husband was gentle and kind and really wanted me to feel pleasure that I began to enjoy sex. Before, I just went through the motions and wanted it to be over."

Do you know how many women tell me that sex is merely "going through the motions"? Thousands! Which means that thousands of women think of sex as routine, boring, one-sided, and/or painful. The bottom line is this: too many women are not enjoying sex. This in turn means that they are uninvolved or disconnected from their sexual experience. This kind of detachment occurs for many reasons. Some women withdraw from their partners because they are angry or hurt, or both. Some women withdraw because sexual intimacy makes them feel too vulnerable. This type of reaction is usually related to a painful or traumatic situation in the past, which for many women can have a lasting impact that closes them off from sex psychologically, emotionally, and physically.

My point? That by becoming aware of and understanding

our early sexual experiences—positive or negative—we give ourselves the opportunity to update our view of ourselves. If your
first sexual experience was unpleasant, that shouldn't mean sex has
to remain an unpleasant part of your life. Far from it. By understanding what happened in the past and how you'd like things
to be different today and in the future, you can change your experience. If, on the other hand, your early experiences with sex were
positive, that's fantastic! But you can still learn more—and enjoy
more—by exploring your sexual self. Do you really want to
go through life missing out on such an important part of who
you are?

These questions are also asking you to be honest about where
you are now in terms of your sexuality. If you are in a relationship,
are you happy, satisfied, and well taken care of sexually? If your
response was a quick and easy "yes," then get ready to discover
many new ways to enhance your intimacy with your partner. If,
however, you hesitated to respond, or if a resounding "no!" echoed
in your ears, then you need to acknowledge the truth about your
situation and consider what you can change. I remember one evening at the end of a Pure Romance party, when fifty-two-year old
Connie finally reached her own breaking point. All evening, she
had been the life of the party, entertaining the other women with
the stories about how much her husband wants her all the time.
But as soon as she came into the confidential Ordering Room, she
broke down in front of me and started sobbing. Despite her bra-
vado and big personality, Connie was miserable.

"You don't know what my life is like," she cried.

"So tell me," I encouraged her.

"My husband has no interest in me at all," she said. "We never
have sex."

It was clear that Connie had put up a charade to cover her pain and disappointment in her husband and her marriage. I suggested that she buy some products for herself first. Before she could figure out what she could change in her relationship, she needed to take responsibility for herself, and that included reconnecting with her sexual self. (You will find more information on what bedroom accessories are right for you in Chapter 8.)

This is often the first step to finding your sexual comfort zone. We tend to jump too fast to "save" or "fix" our relationship, when what we really need is to get back on track with ourselves. Another story comes to mind. This situation took place at an end-of-the-year Pure Romance party back in the early days when I felt a lot of pressure to sell products. I was a single mom with four growing kids and the financial pressure was on. In the confidential Ordering Room, Gail, a pretty, thirty-something woman, ordered an array of products—pretty much one of everything. From a sales perspective I was thrilled.

As I filled in her information, we began talking and I asked Gail if she was planning an anniversary or some special surprise for her husband. She nodded a bit shyly and then told me her story: a few months back, she was desperate to try and fix her relationship. Her husband had mentioned a fantasy he had about having a threesome. Instead of taking that as a signal that they should begin thinking outside of the box and find new ways to spice up their relationship, Gail took the fantasy literally and felt that by doing something a bit "outrageous," she and her husband might re-find the sexual spark between them, so she arranged a threesome with her best friend and her husband at a cabin in the woods.

Unfortunately, the only outrageous thing that happened was that her husband and her girlfriend began their own private affair.

Now, Gail was trying woo her husband back by wowing him with some bedroom accessories.

"What have I done?" she said.

I looked at her and said, "Do you want to try these products?" When she hesitated and then explained she was doing it "for her husband," I scooped up all the items on the table and said, "I don't want you to buy these. They are not going to save your marriage. Why don't you buy a couple of things for yourself and take the money and spend it on professional help for you and your husband."

Although a part of me was sad to see a big sale go by, it was more important to me that Gail understood what had happened. She had moved out of her comfort zone and not only didn't help her relationship but undermined herself. So as you consider where you are now in your relationship or within yourself, think about what is right for you—and never undermine or betray yourself.

If you have ever been victimized or traumatized sexually, it's important that you receive the help you need. The American Association of Sexuality Educators, Counselors, and Therapists (AASECT) is a trusted source for finding a therapist or counselor in your area who will help you work through any kind of trauma or abuse. Contact www.aasect.org for more information.

Sex Is an Inside Thing

In my travels, women come up to me asking and sometimes begging for advice on how to turn on their man, how to have simultaneous orgasms, or how to give mind-blowing oral sex. And most of the time, I say, "Okay, but slow down, already!" Sure, great sex and becoming a great lover is about technique. But only partly. It's also about going inside yourself and being fully present. It's about letting yourself become aware of every inch of your body and paying attention to how your body responds to touch, to music, to kissing, to whatever is happening to or around you.

It's hard to tell people how to get inside themselves. When you're having an orgasm, it's about creating a bubble in which you pay attention to what is building and close your eyes so you can appreciate all the feelings. When you're with your partner, it's about feeling his body against your skin, his sweat dripping onto you, and letting yourself get into the sensuality of sex. It's also about giving that same attention to your partner. Are you watching, listening to, and feeling how he responds when you touch him?

Try something right now. Close your eyes and let yourself travel. Imagine yourself on a beach. Can you feel the soft breeze on your face, your arms? Can you feel the sand between your toes? Can you hear the rhythm of the waves as the surf comes in? Can you smell the salty air? If you are able to let your mind travel, and if you are able to imagine the above sensual experiences, then you can certainly bring that same level of attention and heightened awareness to your lovemaking. Having wonderful sex is much more about being fully engaged in what you are doing than it is about any technique you can perform.

This is especially true for women, for whom arousal is much more complex and varied than it is for men (you'll learn more about arousal in the next chapter). Some women conjure up an image of a dream man touching and pleasuring them. Other women create a fantasy map of their bodies, in which they go on a treasure hunt of pleasure, imagining each of their favorite spots being touched or caressed. Some women need something more physical to get them aroused—whether that means touching themselves, using a vibrator, or having their partner touch or stimulate them in a particular way. But regardless of precisely how you get aroused, you need to experience this arousal *inside*—by paying attention with your mind.

Whether or not you're in a relationship, it's important to start with yourself—romance yourself, I like to say. Once you form this bond with yourself, you automatically lay the groundwork for intimacy—first with yourself and then with your partner.

ASK PATTY:
A Small Question

Hello Patty,

I'm kind of embarrassed to ask you this, but I figure you would be best since we don't know each other. I am a twenty-five-year-old female and I don't know whether or not I've climaxed, reached the big "O", or experienced this so-called out-of-body feeling. Numerous people say I need to start masturbating to figure out what it takes and how it feels. However, I've had partners who have told me that I have climaxed, and I've seen the puddles/ejaculation from myself. But I have never felt that out-of-body, earth-shattering feeling. Do you think I'm looking too much into it, or expecting too much from an orgasm? If anything, can you recommend a toy that will help me masturbate & orgasm? I've never really done it before, but I'm trying to overcome my insecurities about it.

Thank you!

Dear Small Question:

First of all, if you don't think you've had an orgasm, then you probably haven't. But more importantly, it's up to you to decide and define your own sexual experience. Just because a partner tells you that you've climaxed doesn't mean it's true.

Your girlfriends are probably right: masturbation is a private way for you to learn more about yourself. Find a quiet, safe time and place and experiment with a vibrator or bullet. One of the best ways to learn to orgasm is through self-pleasuring, which is not only a completely personal way to get to know yourself, it can also be enormously satisfying. I can't stress to you enough that you define your own sexual experience—orgasm or not.

Truly,
Patty

Change Is Everything

Sex changes. We change. Relationships change. Our bodies change. If we don't accept this fact of life, then we set ourselves up for unrealistic expectations in all areas of our lives. The women I work with who have the most difficulty finding—or refinding—their comfort zone are usually struggling with change: They need to remain open to change and be ready for it one way or another. Amy is one of my favorite product vendors and a woman I consider one of my closest friends. She was widowed about five years ago when her husband died of a brain tumor. During a girlfriends' weekend in Miami, I asked her, "So have you begun dating?"

She shook her head no, and said, "I just can't even wrap my head around it. I don't think enough time has passed."

Deciding when you are ready to resume dating is an entirely personal decision, but I did want to start talking about intimacy issues.

So I said, "You're telling me you haven't had any sex or penetration?"

"No," she said.

"Well, did you know that if you don't use it, you might just lose it?" I asked her gently.

Amy looked shocked. Here was a woman who thought she knew everything there was to know about her sexuality, and yet she didn't really understand that her sexual plumbing, so to speak, could stop functioning from mere lack of use. Essentially if a woman goes too long without using her sexual muscles (more on this later!) or being sexually active—either with a partner or on her own—then her vaginal walls can literally collapse, causing not only pain but an inability to become aroused or orgasm.

It was clear to me that it would take more time before Amy felt ready to date again. But I sent her a bedroom toy with some heartfelt suggestions on how being intimate with herself could really benefit her body and her mind. She called me a few weeks later, saying, "I not only owe you at least three dinners the next time we get together, I owe you so much more—I feel alive again!"

We know our bodies change day to day, month to month, year to year. What we often are not aware of is how these changes impact our sexuality. Amy was still a vibrant woman in her early fifties. Did she want to sacrifice her sexuality for the rest of her days? Not on her life. But she needed some gentle encouragement and some knowledge.

It's Up to You

Finding your comfort zone about sex is also about knowing your boundaries and limits. Never let anyone pressure you to do or try something that makes you feel uncomfortable. And don't let a partner make you feel guilty—sex is something to engage in respectfully.

When we stay open to learning about sex, ourselves, and our partners, we allow for wonderful, magical possibilities. At its most basic level, sex is about pleasure and release. It's not about taking notes or memorizing techniques. It's about getting to know yourself, paying attention, and then following your intuition—wherever that may lead!

Sexuality is a *big* part of who we are as human beings. It's written into our DNA, it's a driving force, and it can be a source of enormous pleasure. If this part of you is not nurtured and stimulated, your health suffers—there are mental, emotional, and physical consequences to denying or suppressing your sexuality. So let's throw outdated, harmful myths right out the window! Being a sexually active, aware woman does not mean that you are "bad" or "naughty"—it simply means you are alive.

One of my top consultants loves to say at Pure Romance parties, "I want to save one vagina at a time!" She's not on a mission to make women into sex machines—in fact, quite the opposite. She wants women simply to open up to who they are and to this important, life-sustaining part of themselves. Taking care of your sexuality is the most deeply personal way to take care of yourself—and your relationship—and the bonus is that it can be tons of fun too!

CHAPTER TWO

Your Love, Your Life, Your Libido

"I JUST NEVER FEEL in the mood for sex anymore." "I can't remember the last time I felt excited by even the idea of being intimate with my husband—nothing is going on down there." "Ever since the birth of my first baby, I don't *want* sex—period. We now have three kids, and I just go through the motions. When will I ever feel excited again?"

I have heard literally hundreds—if not thousands—of women say these and similar words to me over the past twenty-five years. What are they referring to? Libido, or sexual desire and how it is missing in their lives. By now, many of us have read or heard about the statistic that an astounding 40 percent of women in this country experience no or very low sexual desire. But what does this number really mean? In some cases, low libido has clear medical causes; but in other cases, the decline or absence of sexual desire stems from a combination of emotional and physiological causes. A lack of libido may be a reaction to a negative past experience that has created a wall between a woman and her ability to feel sexual pleasure. Some women are not experiencing sexual desire because a medication they are taking—from antihistamines to antidepressants—is interfering with how their bodies respond sexually. Other women don't realize their birth control pill (or patch) actually mutes their desire. Who knew feeling in the mood for sex was so complicated?

Whatever the reason—and there are many—experiencing low desire can be very frustrating and confusing. But, ladies, the good news is that in many cases, it is also treatable. Before we take a closer look at why your libido may be inhibited and how to strengthen it, let's take a look at the sexual response cycle and where your libido fits in.

The Sexual Response Cycle: A Bird's-Eye View

Over twenty-five years ago, Masters and Johnson published a now-revolutionary study, *Human Sexual Response*, first defining the sexual response cycle. Somewhat arbitrarily they divided this cycle into four stages:

1. Arousal
2. Plateau
3. Orgasm
4. Resolution

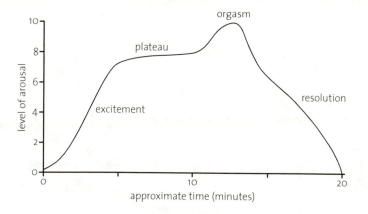

Masters and Johnson's Human Sexual Response Cycle

According to M&J, the cycle begins with arousal (stage 1), which is the body's physical response to sexual excitement. Arousal then plateaus (stage 2), as it builds toward a climax or orgasm (stage 3). Once orgasm is achieved, the body returns to its "normal" preexcited state (resolution, stage 4).

Although this information helped many people, researchers included, understand their sexual experience more clearly, not everyone was able to fit that experience neatly into these four stages. The great sexologist Alfred Kinsey has said, "There is nothing more characteristic of sexual response than the fact that it is not the same in any two individuals." First of all, many people can experience desire, arousal, and satisfaction without experiencing an orgasm. Second, many people—especially women—describe their sexual experience as more subtle and less linear. Since M&J first defined their four stages, many researchers—and many others as well—have described their sexual response cycle in five stages:

1. Desire—an interest in sex

2. Excitement—feeling of arousal

3. Plateau—a consistent level of arousal

4. Orgasm—a sexual climax

5. Resolution—a return to an unexcited state.

In this scenario, the first stage of the cycle begins with a desire for sex, prompting the person to seek a partner or some form of self-pleasuring, which in turn leads to sexual arousal (the body's physical reaction to desire). Arousal (stage 2) enables the body to gradually build in excitement (stage 3), culminating in an orgasm (stage 4). After this climax, the body returns to the unexcited state (resolution, stage 5).

Many women say that the desire for sex often begins more emotionally in their minds—they need to feel comfortable in their own skin, or in sync with their partner. When they feel good emotionally, they can then relax enough to let their bodies get turned on (i.e., aroused). Women also describe the "plateau" as a gradual

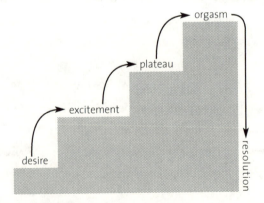

building or meandering of pleasure and excitement. Sometimes this feeling leads to an orgasm; sometimes it does not.

Also, many women actually describe their sexual cycle as being more circular, being able to move through desire and excitement, without ever having to experience orgasm. So if you've ever wondered whether you are "normal," keep in mind that normal is whatever gives you pleasure. Again, many women don't have to reach orgasm to feel a desire for sex or fulfillment from a sexual experience. In other words, we all experience our cycle in very idiosyncratic ways.

Why are these stages important at all? They point to why both libido and arousal are the essential starting points for sexual pleasure, and if you have a problem with either one (or both), you might be experiencing less than your potential in the pleasure department. Now let's take a look at the mysterious libido, and what stimulates our desire for sex.

In the National Health and Social Life Survey, approximately 33 percent of women between eighteen and fifty-nine years of age reported a loss of sexual desire for at least a few months over the last year.

The Libido Triangle

Although nearly 40 percent of women say they don't experience sexual desire, another 50-plus percent do enjoy the pleasure, the satisfaction, and the wonderful way that having an active libido

*Source: *Journal of the American Medical Association*, Volume 292, No. 14

makes them feel alive and in sync with themselves. Carly, a forty-something woman describes libido in a very physical way: "It's the itch, the urge, the need for sex." Michelle, who is younger, in her late twenties, defines libido in more emotional terms: "It's more a mood-thing for me. When I feel really close to my boyfriend—it's like I want to merge with him." And thirty-five-year-old Jacqui said this: "I've always been a sexual person, and I'm thankful for that. It's not like I want sex all the time, it's more that this part of myself grounds me in who I am. It's a reminder that I am a woman." Can you hear the sense of power and confidence in Jacqui's voice?

These women capture the great variability of how women experience their libido. But what is happening when there's a problem? Historically, the term libido was coined by the founder of psychoanalysis, Sigmund Freud, who defined it as a sexual "drive" or "instinct." And while Freud's work contributed to identifying and questioning the mere existence of female sexuality, many of his ideas definitely missed the mark. (For instance, he felt that clitoral orgasm was an "immature" orgasm—think again, Dr. Freud.) But my point is that libido or sexual desire is a somewhat amorphous concept. It refers sometimes to a physical hunger or need for sex (body), or it speaks to a woman's way of becoming interested in or excited by sex (mind). Or it may relate more to a woman's connection with herself or her lover (heart). The most all-encompassing way to approach your libido is the idea of a libido triangle, made up of three sources of desire that point to a woman's body, mind, and/or heart. When you think of libido as stemming from one or all three of these points, you can understand your own libido on your own terms, in whatever way is most natural to you.

However, if one or all of these points on a woman's libido triangle are not stimulated or engaged, she will simply not feel like having sex. Her body won't "feel the urge"; her mind will feel "disengaged"; and her heart will feel closed off, as if a ten-foot wall surrounds it. In talking to women and responding to countless questions about how to help them with low or no sexual desire, I have found that feeling interested in sex depends on many factors. Women say they need to:

"feel in the mood for sex"

"feel connected to their partner"

"feel loved and cherished by their partner"

"feel attractive, sexy, or desirable"

"feel wanted or desired by their partner"

"have a romantic environment"

And while this is what women say, what scientists and sex-ologists have shown to be true in their research is that libido depends on:

♡ An ability to become aroused

♡ A healthy attitude toward sex

♡ Proper sexual functioning

So when a woman is not experiencing libido or has noticed a loss of desire, one of these three components has more than likely been impacted. In medical or scientific terms, doctors and sexolo-gists say that problems with libido are either *medical* (i.e., an infection or a side effect from medication is impacting libido); *physiological* (i.e., some kind of interplay between hormones, pain or irritation, or diet that has interfered with a woman's ability to feel pleasure and by extension has muted her libido); or *psychosocial* (i.e., causes that are related to cultural or religious views about sex, some kind of traumatic or negative experience or abuse, or situational stress or anxiety that may be inhibit libido).* No wonder so many women say they don't feel like having sex!

Libido vs. Arousability

So what happens when we become aroused? Perhaps a woman is stimulated through kissing or touching of her breasts; this stimulation then triggers blood flow to the pelvis, stimulating the labia, clitoris, and the pubococcygeus (PC) muscles. The vagina itself moistens, the lips begin to swell, and lubrication increases. For many women, lubrication is one of the first signs of sexual arousal. Physiologically, lubrication corresponds to an erection for men, yet women often take much longer to lubricate than men take to get an erection. Women's bodies will naturally respond as they were designed to during arousal, but often men will seem to be way ahead of them—a man may be erect and ready to go while the woman is still getting warmed up. Although some women will begin to lubricate within thirty seconds of being stimulated—either mentally or physically—not all women do. Some may take several minutes or not lubricate at all, and this may be one of the first triggers that inhibits libido down the road. (You will find a

* Source: The Women's Sexual Health Foundation, www.twshf.org

further discussion for vaginal dryness and inability or difficulty with lubrication in Chapter 3.)

So how can you help yourself become aroused? Researchers at the University of Amsterdam recently looked at how women experience sexual desire and found that it might just be more effective to focus on enhancing arousability rather than desire, since arousal is more concrete and tangible. Again, since women respond to many different stimuli—some of it mental, some more emotional, and some purely physical—you need to figure out what triggers *your* arousal. As thirty-something Kate said, "The only way I get aroused enough to be sexual with my husband is if I first touch myself." This is true of many women, who need direct clitoral stimulation in order to become aroused. Dana, who is in her early fifties, says, "For me to get that feeling between my legs, I have to fantasize. I think of really intense encounters that have happened in the past—I have a few favorites—and that's what gets me hot. Otherwise, I think it would be really hard—I've been with my husband for over twenty years!"

Both Kate and Dana know exactly what they need to get turned on, but in completely different ways. For Kate, it's something physical; for Dana, it's something more mental. Regardless of the relationship between libido (desire) and arousal, you need to figure out what gets you excited. Which leads me to my next question: what turns you on?

Before you even try to answer that question, keep in mind four things:

1. There is no right or wrong answer to that question.
2. There may be many answers to that question.

3. Your answer may change, depending on your mood, the time of the month, your age, or even who you are with.

4. You may not know the answer to that question . . . yet!

Thankfully, there are a number of ways to get in touch with how you become aroused, and as a result boost your libido. And they all have to do with getting to know yourself better, starting with your body.

Intimacy Issue #2—"I have no desire for sex."

We've been hearing a lot about how millions of women have no desire for sex. I'd like to turn this statistic on its head! Just like Deirdre, a twenty-year-old college sophomore, Elaine, a thirty-seven-year-old stay-at-home mom, and Zale, a fiftyish divorced woman, you can move from no desire to great desire. The more you understand the connection between your body and your libido, and your mind and your arousability, the more in control of your sexuality you will become. Low libido is not the end; it's only the beginning. And it's my sincere belief that with more information and more understanding, women will feel more confident and in control of what may always have been a vast unknown area.

Keep in mind, too, that it's truly up to you to know what turns you on. When women come into the Ordering Room and complain, "My partner does not know what he's doing—he's just a bad lover!" I always remind them that men are not born knowing how to please us and we were not born knowing what gives us pleasure. You need to start by discovering your own path to sensation, and then you can begin to communicate this to your partner. Consider the tips on self-pleasuring and exploring how you enjoy being stimulated. This is the first and best step to tapping into your libido. If you still need help, try one of our arousal creams (see page 61 for more information). Although some women cannot physiologically experience sexual desire, most of us can—so try not to give up hope.

Anatomy Lesson—A Guide to Your Intimate Parts

You may think you know where everything is "down there," but let's just take time for a bit of a refresher. Take a look at the illustration. Familiarize yourself with its details.

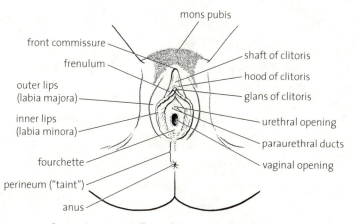

Source: American College of Obstetrics and Gynecology

Some Vaginal Surprises

Did you know that

♡ your labia majora (the large lips that surround the vaginal opening) and the labia minora (the thinner, inner lips, which have no hair follicles) fill with blood during arousal, causing them to swell and stiffen?

♡ only a small part of your clitoris is actually visible? The "legs" of this sensitive structure extend all the way back along the roof of the vagina.

♡ over 65 percent of women need direct clitoral stimulation for orgasm?

♡ there are over eight thousand nerve endings in the clitoris?

♡ many women experience a lot of pleasure from stimulation of the perineum, the very sensitive spot between the anus and the entry of the vagina?

♡ your g-spot is under the skin of the roof of your vagina and can only be felt when stimulated?

♡ your g-spot actually grows from the size of a dime to the size of a walnut when stimulated?

♡ the muscles that control your orgasm are the same ones that control the flow of urine? Your pubococcygeus muscle or PC muscle is a hammock-like muscle that stretches from the pubic bone to the coccyx (the tail bone), forming the floor of your pelvis. These important muscles not only enable

bladder control, labor, and childbirth, but are crucial to proper sexual functioning and ability to feel
pleasure. When these muscles are kept toned and
strong, you increase your ability to become aroused
with clitoral stimulation and experience a vaginal
orgasm. (See Chapter 4 for more information on
how to strengthen and tone these muscles.)

Self-Pleasuring

Why is it important for you to know your anatomy? Well, for one
thing, don't you want to know what you or your partner is touching? The more familiar you are with how your body works, the
more likely you will be able to zero in on exactly what kind of
touching feels good. On the other hand, if you are experiencing
pain or discomfort, you will be better able to pinpoint the source
of the pain. So another important way to find out what turns you
on is by getting to know yourself more intimately.

Remember when our mothers wagged their fingers or told us
not to touch ourselves? Those are bygone days. We are now women
who want and have the right to know exactly how our bodies
work and how they respond to touch and pleasurable stimulation.
Do you know how many women don't even know where their
clitoris is? We can never start too early, or too late. Just recently, a
woman approached me after a presentation and said, "I know I
should be comfortable with masturbation, but I can't get my
mother's voice out of my head telling me not to touch myself.
What can I do to be more relaxed?" This is a very common question: women want to discover more pleasure, but are held back by

old attitudes that make them think of masturbation as "dirty" or "improper." Being able to be sensual with yourself is a very private, intimate experience. It's about you and only you. Some women use their special time when they are in the shower or bath; they use waterproof bedroom toys or even the shower head to begin to explore their bodies and what feels good. I always suggest investing in a vibrator—some women are not comfortable with using their hands.

The idea is to relax and let yourself touch your body—not just your genitals but your breasts, your abdomen, and even your arms. You need to make a decision about what's right for you. Maybe you will enjoy watching soft porn or reading some erotica or a romance novel. Sometimes you need something that arouses you or triggers your body. Play soft music. Light a scented candle, put on a soft, luxurious bathrobe after a shower. Romance yourself. You need to pay attention to how your body feels as you become more sensually aware and tuned into sensation. And, as always, there is no right or wrong way to self-pleasuring—there's just your way.

As our largest organ, our skin can provide an endless source of pleasure, even if this pleasure is more sensual than sexual in nature. For wonderful, female positive advice on how to masturbate and become comfortable exploring self-pleasuring, there is no better source than Betty Dodson's classic book *Sex for One*. And in Chapter 8 of this book you will find great ways to investigate the kind of touching that you find arousing by using vibrators, dildos, and other bedroom accessories that enhance pleasure. Without a doubt, one of the fastest and easiest ways a woman can discover sexual pleasure is with the bullet (a small vibrator). For generations, this simple instrument has helped millions of women get in touch with themselves, which is why the bullet tends to be the most popular toy.

Your Hormones and Libido

We hear a lot about our hormones ruling our bodies, but did you know that they also impact our libido? Stacy, who I first met at a party before she went on to become a consultant herself, is a passionate woman who said she had always had a strong sexual libido and a great sex life with her husband of eighteen years. But at forty-five, Stacy suddenly was finding all sorts of excuses for avoiding sex with her husband.

After hearing her story, I suggested that she visit her ob-gyn to see if her hormones were playing a role in her sudden loss of libido. With her doctor's help, Stacy determined that she was perimenopausal and her body had begun to produce both less estrogen and less testosterone, the main two hormones related to libido.

As women age, it's perfectly natural to produce less estrogen and testosterone, but it doesn't mean you have to say good-bye to your libido. Some women consult their doctors and get hormonal replacement therapy (HRT); others find more temporary ways to increase their libido, including arousal creams (for more information on arousal creams, see page 61). As for Stacy, she invested in an arousal cream and also began to pay more attention to what got her in the mood for sex. When I spoke to her again a few months later, she and her husband were back on track, enjoying being intimate together and feeling so much more connected.

Another way our hormones can impact our libido is through birth control pills (or the patch), which suppress ovulation (in order to prevent pregnancy) by consistently raising estrogen. Margaret, at twenty-five, had gone on birth control when she became more seriously involved with her boyfriend. "I was ready to go on a more consistent form of birth control, but I didn't know my desire for sex was going to go out the window."

Many young women are surprised by this connection, but it's true. Of course, some women still experience an adequate libido on the pill and prefer this method of putting off pregnancy. But if you are concerned about your loss of libido as it relates to the pill, you should consult your physician or health care provider for other forms of birth control that don't impact your hormones.

In the next chapter, you will learn more in-depth information about how your hormones can impact your libido and your overall sexual functioning. But suffice it to say that there are two major ways that your hormones can impact your libido:

♡ Birth control pills (or the patch)
♡ Natural effects of aging when your body produces less estrogen and testosterone

The good news is that currently, more and more doctors and health care providers are looking at safe and effective ways to address these side effects so women can continue to feel sexually vital into their sixties and beyond!

Dear Patty,

Is it possible that birth control pills can have an effect on my sexual drive? I have noticed a decreasing sex drive over the past year and the only thing that I can relate it to is that I began taking birth control a little more than a year ago.

Thanks.

Anonymous

Dear Anonymous,

While reducing your sex drive is certainly a form of birth control, it is probably not the type of control we typically think of (or want) when deciding to use oral contraceptives. The answer to your question is: Yes. The pill does affect some women's sex drive. The good news is, if a particular pill has negative side effects, there are a number of other pills to try. Birth control pills come in several different forms. The most common are the combined oral contraceptives, a mixture of estrogen and progestin.

Talk to your doctor or nurse practitioner about switching pills. If you are currently on a combined pill, look for one with a different amount of progestin, or try a progestin-only pill. Be aware that the progestin-only pills may cause spot bleeding and irregular periods—not a medical problem, but possibly an annoyance.

There are other ways to enhance your sex drive if it has been inhibited by the use of birth control pills. Increasing the use of some of our foreplay items, such as Dust Me Pink or Sinfully Sweet, or using heighteners or arousal creams, such as Ex-T-Cee, can really enhance the level of sexual excitement you are experiencing during intercourse. It is important to communicate with your partner and discuss where you think the problem is occurring. Maybe simply adding a lubricant to your routine will spice things up and increase your level of arousal, or maybe changing your birth control pill is what it will take to improve your sex drive.

You may be interested to know that Indiana University's Kinsey Institute for Research in Sex, Gender and Reproduction is currently studying the effects of birth control pills on mood and sexuality. We hope this information will help women make informed decisions about the right pill for them.

I hope this was helpful!

Truly,
Patty

Other Medicines that Inhibit Libido

When I travel the country speaking to college students on their campuses, I am always surprised by how many students complain of having no or low sex drive. Nine times out of ten, the reason is some kind of medication they are taking that they didn't know was lessening their libido. As I've said, the two main medications that can interrupt libido are antidepressants and antihistamines. I've said I often begin a college talk by asking if students know the connection between having a cold and becoming dry in all their orifices. The connection is based on the common way to treat a cold or the flu: by taking an antihistamine, which dries up all of our orifices, including those in our genitals.

It is important to point out that some commonly used medications can inhibit sexual desire. Most common are the new antidepressants such as fluoxetine (Prozac), sertraline (Zoloft), and paroxetine (Paxil). These may decrease sexual desire and performance in up to a fifth of people taking them. Sometimes they simply slow response so it takes longer to become aroused and longer to attain orgasm. Antidepressants can have these effects in both women and men, and only one, bupropion (Wellbutrin) doesn't have a libido-lowering impact. In fact, some people say they have experienced an increase in their libido on Wellbutrin. Blood pressure medicines, cholesterol-lowering medications, antihistamines, and some antipsychotic drugs can also interfere with libido. (A complete list of medications that impact desire and arousal can be found in the Resources section.)

ASK PATTY:
No Desire Anymore

Dear Patty,

I am only twenty-four and I really just don't want to have sex anymore. I think this is a problem, because my husband always wants to be intimate with me. I really don't know what it is, but lately I just don't have the desire anymore. I have always had a high sex drive even after two kids. I love him very much, but I am afraid this is going to be a big problem for us. What should I do?

Lost and in Love

Dear Lost and in Love,

There are a lot of women out there who can relate to your situation. Your intimate life can be a lot like a roller coaster. It can have its peaks, but it can also have its dips. I feel for you, but the good thing is, we are here to help. Our society often confuses the definitions of love, intimacy, and sex, and furthermore, draws a conclusion that you must have one to have the other.

Well, we think they are wrong. Although you might still love your husband, it is often hard to find time to engage in passionate sex—or even just sex—when you have kids and laundry and not enough energy to do one more thing. But the fact of the matter is that you are responsible for creating satisfaction in the bedroom ultimately through effort and communication to your partner . . . it's time you found the energy to put into your intimate relationship with your husband for you, him, and even your kids.

My first suggestion to you is to talk to your husband. Communication is the key to happiness. Since most of us sometimes forget the basics in communication, play a game. We have several games (i.e., Card Game for Lovers) that can help you open up the lines of communication, and get passionate again. Chances are if you have lost communication in the bedroom, you have probably lost touch in other aspects of your life. You might be surprised at how receptive he is to your concerns. Just think, he is probably as eager as you are to nip this in the bud!

After you talk to your husband, try to make an effort to reconnect with him emotionally. Find out what's going on in his life. Ask him what his favorite color is. Just because it was blue when you first met doesn't mean it will be the same forever. People change as they grow and part of being in an evolving relationship is being able to learn about each other as you grow. You don't want to make the mistake of thinking your partner will always have the same likes, dislikes, and interests as he or she did when you first began getting to know each other. Set aside time each day to just talk. Once you have reconnected emotionally, it will be much easier to start the process to reconnect physically.

Now, you mentioned kids. Don't hesitate to schedule a date night, babysitter and all! Once you have some alone time, start out by just physically touching one another. A massage might be the perfect start to a fulfilling sexual relationship.

When you are ready to have intercourse again I would recommend using an arousal cream. You will place a small pea-sized amount on your clitoris a few minutes before intercourse. It causes the blood to rush to that area creating a heightened sensitivity. Mentally it allows your brain to forget everything else

*and focus on what feels good and allow you to act
on it. And don't forget your gentle, water-based lubricant!*

*Just remember to place your focus on the intimate
aspects of your relationship, such as communication,
massage, hugging and cuddling and put your mind
on the most important thing, each other.*

Truly, Patty

Looking in the Mirror

Jill was a forty-eight-year-old mother of twins, whom she had just sent off to college. "Suddenly, it's just me and my husband." She described her sex life as "mediocre," but told me that she loved her husband very much. "I guess I think about myself as not very sexual—I thought that was just how I am." When we began to talk and review her lifestyle and her attitudes about sex, it became clear that Jill had simply never made sex a priority in her life. But now she was a young empty-nester with time on her hands. "I want to make this time in my marriage special—we had our family so young and my husband and I have worked so hard for so long. Now we want to enjoy ourselves." We discussed her options, and how she really needed to get reacquainted with herself first, and then turn to her relationship. A few weeks after she bought some products, she wrote me an email: "I feel like a new person. Suddenly, I feel like a sensual woman—I can't believe what I've been missing!"

Many times, your libido is not low, it's simply missing. And once you take a good look at yourself, and become reacquainted with that person in the mirror, you can—and will—rediscover your sex drive. However, sometimes, looking in the mirror means overcoming a deeper, more hidden part of yourself.

In Chapter 1, I asked you to think about your early sexual experiences so that you could get in touch with who you are as a sexual person and so that you could bring to mind any sexual encounter or event that might have caused you pain or hurt—either emotionally or physically. Any kind of trauma or abuse can have a drastic or significant negative impact on your libido. Many women have been raised in families where sex was associated with judgment, shame, and other negative feelings. And while a woman may grow up thinking she has left these "outdated" views at home in her parent's basement, a negative belief system found in a conservative family or one that has a negative or restrictive view about sex can making a lasting and lingering impact on how women think and feel about sex.

Sandy had contacted me in hopes that I might help her "feel more sexual." She told me that she and her husband Michael were in love, but she often found herself pretending to be turned on when they had sex. Sandy indicated that she truly wanted to feel sexual, but she "just couldn't." She wasn't on any medication that would be interfering; and she wasn't on the pill—in fact, she and Michael were trying to get pregnant. There seemed to be no medical or hormonal issue going on. So I suspected that Sandy was probably suffering from some kind of emotional block. I began by asking Sandy about her past. She had grown up in a strict, conservative household, and she was taught that sex was only for reproduction. This was not so unusual, and I continued to dig a bit deeper. It turned out that as a fifteen-year-old, Sandy had been molested by an older cousin. So mortified by this experience, she was embarrassed to tell her parents for fear that they would reject her. Now, age twenty-five, Sandy was still carrying around this shame—as if she wasn't a victim of abuse but rather the perpetrator!

Any kind of sexual molestation, abuse, or negative sexual experience can have a profound effect on how a woman, especially a young woman, experiences her sexuality. Feelings of guilt, shame, and despair are difficult to unravel and resolve, but not insurmountable. And when women refuse to give up on their right to enjoy and be proud of their sexuality, they empower themselves.

If you have ever been forced to do something you didn't want to do, you will more than likely carry this forward into your new relationship unless you make a conscious effort to resolve it. (Often this takes some kind of professional help.) Unfortunately many women have been abused or traumatized sexually. It makes my heart cringe every time I hear about an experience such as Sandy's. For some women (and men), these wounds never seem to heal, but the good news is that many people have successfully dealt with their emotional injuries and reclaimed their sensuality and sexuality. If you are struggling with abuse or traumas, don't give up. There are many skilled practitioners who can help. And if you have found a loving partner, he or she may be eager to help heal these wounds and very much want to be the one who brings back your sexual delight and desire.

If you—or anyone you know or love—has ever experienced a sexual trauma, it's very important to seek out counseling and/or professional help. AASECT provides a reliable source of counselors and treatment options in your area.

What You Can Do to Enhance Your Libido

Although in the next chapter I go into more detail about the causes for the loss of libido and difficulty with sexual responsiveness, you may be wondering what you can do to enhance or trigger your libido. Again, the place to start is by learning more about your own body and how it responds to sensual and sexual stimulation. Beyond that, there are both direct and indirect ways, including arousal creams, diet, and targeted exercises.

Arousal Creams

A powerful and immediate way to help boost libido and increase arousability is through heighteners, or arousal creams. When applied directly on the genitalia, a heightener is designed to make the clitoris engorge with blood and the tissue more sensitive. The use of a heightener can help intensify genital sensitivity in both men and women, enhancing sexual pleasure and the possibility of orgasm. Talk about getting you in the mood fast!

I always say that arousal creams are a great way to level the playing field for women because they help them feel more aroused even when they are not as mentally into having sex. Arousal creams bypass the brain and cause blood to rush to the genital area much faster. At Pure Romance, we offer an array of such products that have different uses. For example, Ex-T-Cee is a wonderfully flavored cream whose natural mint ingredients provide a "tingling" sensation to the genitals. It comes in different flavors and contains special sensitizers for women, intensifying feeling in the erogenous zones. Nympho Niagra is an all-natural balm that increases sexual response in a more sensitive way. It is colorless, odorless, and has no flavor, making it a logical choice for women who are prone to yeast and urinary tract infections. This heightener is designed for women who have a low sex drive due to stress, exhaustion, or medication, like birth control pills.

X-Scream is an edible, air-activated unisex heightener that is recommended for women or men experiencing difficulties during arousal. It has a higher concentration of active ingredients than Ex-T-Cee, which creates a more intense stimulating effect. This heightener is great for men or women with an extremely low sex drive or who suffer from the sexual side effects of many medications, particularly antianxiety and antidepressants. (Visit www .pureromance.com for more information.)

Each woman is different in terms of her sexuality and what she finds pleasurable, so we offer a variety of heighteners to meet every woman's needs. Choose the one that sounds most appropriate to your sexual needs and enjoy!

However, if you are having trouble becoming aroused or are experiencing low libido because of stress, anxiety, or a negative or traumatic experience, you may still need to address those issues in addition to using a heightener.

Food for Thought

In order to give our bodies the best opportunity to respond sexually, including triggering libido and enhancing arousal, it's important to take care of them—from what we put in our mouths to how much we exercise and pay attention to other lifestyle habits that may actually hamper our libido. Did you know, for instance, that too much sugar and starchy carbohydrates actually lessen libido? Did you know caffeine and smoking can take away from your ability to become aroused?

All of us have busy schedules filled with responsibilities and obligations, and it's often hard to eat right and take the time to exercise. We grab lunch at a fast food restaurant; we skip our trip to the gym—some of us even smoke a cigarette when we are feeling stressed. All of these less-than-good habits impact our sexuality. Renowned sexologist David M. Ferguson, Ph.D., M.D., and president of the Women's Sexual Health Foundation, has pointed out that "large numbers of working people eat 'fast foods' for lunch every day. Labels show these foods also are very high in fats and cereal-based carbohydrates. The result is flavorless nutritionally deficient produce. . . . For sexual responsiveness, the body needs proteins and certain fats while avoiding excess carbohydrates." More to the point, gynecologist and author Rebecca Booth, M.D., points out that "women who don't ovulate regularly . . . will also exhibit a loss of libido," because libido is tied again to a woman's hormonal cycle. Dr. Booth also notes that a common cause of irregular ovulation is too much "white food" in the diet. In fact, the same diet that can cause diabetes, one made up primarily of starchy carbs, white sugar, and not enough fiber, has also been shown to dampen libido.

But the good news is that with a few simple changes, you can actually enhance your libido. Marrena Lindberg, author of *The Orgasmic Diet*, suggests taking fish oil supplements, eating dark chocolate (half an ounce per day), and staying away from starchy carbs and too much unrefined sugar.

So my advice is to look at what you eat. A lot of junk food? Sugar? Have you noticed you are not ovulating or experiencing that peak in your libido midway through your cycle? You may unknowingly be impacting your libido.

Putting It All Together

A lot of factors can contribute to a low sex drive. One of the first things I recommend is taking a general look at your lifestyle. Are you tired all the time and not getting enough sleep? Is there a baby or child in your bed? Being fatigued can lower sex drive. Another significant reason that libido gets muted is stress, something most of us have far too much of in our lives. One woman wrote to me with this story:

"I just got married in June and neither my husband nor I have had very much sex before the wedding. Once we got married, it happened more often, but now there seems to be some problems. My husband is twenty-five and I am twenty-one and it seems his drive isn't quite what mine is. I am hoping it is just because he works a lot, but I feel awkward because I am somewhat like the 'guy' of the relationship."

A couple of things are going on in this woman's situation. First, it seems that her husband's working so much has interfered with his sex drive. And second, she feels uncomfortable that she has more desire than he does, as if her desire makes her more like a "guy" and less like a woman. We all work too much, right? There is always more work to be done; longer hours we could put in. It's very difficult to maintain a good balance between work and downtime—whether you work in an office, your own business, or your job is feeding and taking care of one or ten kids. The bottom line is that work makes us tired and stressed, two big factors that inhibit or mute libido. At the end of the day, you're physically and mentally tired, and all you want to do is relax on the couch. While this is a perfectly understandable reaction, what may begin as a temporary situation can often lead to a more gradual, never-ending pattern, resulting in sex once a month . . . or once a year. So my advice here is: make the time. Your sex life, your connection with your partner, and your health are all too important to put off.

And who said the person in charge of initiating sex has to be the man in the relationship?! One of the first things I share with young women when I do the Pure Romance Naked Truth College Tours is how important it is for them to "own" their sexuality. Not only should they take responsibility for their sexual decisions and sexual health, but they should make their sexuality something important in their lives. So ladies, let me say this loud and clear: if you want to have sex, celebrate that desire. Of course, choose your partner wisely, make sure you feel safe and well respected, but go ahead and act on that libido of yours! When women learn to heighten their libido and tap into what gets them aroused, they become not just more satisfied lovers but more confident women.

CHAPTER THREE

Beyond the Bedroom

Taking Responsibility for Your Sexual Health

A T THE BEGINNING of my career, I made it a point to read every book I could find on women's sexuality. This way, when I described a product to a potential client, I could also explain how that bedroom accessory or lubricant worked in the context of her body. Then, when I started my own company (first Slumber Parties and later Pure Romance), and began receiving so many questions not only about the products but also about sexual health issues such as pain, low libido, and so on, I realized that most women—no matter where they lived or how much money or education they had—had very little access to accurate, complete information about their sexual health. This lack of reliable resources is exactly what motivated me to develop the Sexual Health Education Department of Pure Romance, as well as the Patty Brisben Foundation. Since I am not a doctor or a sexologist, I wanted to be able to point my clients and customers to a place where they could find reliable answers to their questions.

So now, a big part of what I do every day is help women understand their bodies and pay attention to their sexual health. The

Health Education Department is devoted to accessing and delivering the most up-to-date information about health issues impacting women's sexuality. We are dedicated to educating women to be able to make informed decisions about their sexuality by providing an opportunity to safely explore and understand their sexuality, gain confidence in their relationships with themselves and others, and help them gain insight into who they are as sexual beings. In addition, we support ongoing research in women's sexual health, and are affiliated with Indiana University's Center for Sexual Health Promotion, the American Association of Sexuality Educators, Counselors and Therapists (AASECT), and other medical, scientific, and sexual health researchers and educators so that we can continue to support women in their right to find accurate, cutting-edge, and practical information to better their sexual health.

Colleen's Story

Let me share with you a story about how a simple misstep such as not reaching for a bit of lubrication, coupled with a health care system unfamiliar with sexual health issues, led to a profound medical and emotional trauma for one young woman.

Colleen is an astute and thoughtful counselor and educator; she is also a survivor of a trauma related to her sexual health. As she told me,

> I was a naive twenty-one-year-old when my life was forever changed. I was just coming home from a weekend with a friend whose father was losing his battle to cancer.

My boyfriend at the time and I had been dating for almost two years and we had a pretty typical college relationship. He picked me up from the airport and took me home so I could shower and change before we grabbed some dinner. He, like many other men his age, was excited to see me for more than one reason. I had barely gotten out of the shower before he was making his move. To say that I wasn't in the mood is an understatement, but I did what most girls (unfortunately) do and I had sex anyway. I was not aroused and my body had not prepared itself to be intimate. Before I knew it, his skin had stuck to mine and somehow tore my inner and outer labia apart. What I didn't realize was the severity of the issue.

When she arrived at the hospital, Colleen was placed on a gurney, her legs were raised in stirrups, and she was barely secluded in the ER. "I was a complete spectacle—with no privacy and all the medical staff coming in to gawk at me," Colleen remembers. After one doctor told Colleen that she didn't know how to treat her injury, an ob-gyn was called in. In a hurried, almost hostile manner, that doctor proceeded to stitch her labia without administering sufficient pain medication. Colleen returned a week or so later to have the stitches removed, only to go through another round of tortuous pain.

The ob-gyn came into the room and was examining me before I knew what hit me. Then as quickly as that began to happen, he was removing my stitches and the pain started all over again. I started crying and begging him to stop. Thankfully, the nurse stepped in and told the doctor she would take care of my stitches and he would have time to make his next appointment. He left without a word and the nurse sat down next to me. She told me she was going to take as much time as I needed to get through removing my stitches. She applied a numbing cream to the area and would wait a few minutes before trying to remove a stitch. If it hurt, she would apply more cream, wait a few minutes, and try again. We did this for forty-five minutes until the cream began to work effectively enough for the stitches to come out comfortably. She was such a blessing that day. She said that removing the stitches would help it to heal faster. She told me my genitals may never look the same again and if I was worried about it I might want to consider another surgery. No way! I would just have to come to terms with they way I looked now.

But as Colleen pointed out, "that was only the beginning."

I left his office feeling like my world had just changed, and it had. The next couple of months were really rough. My boyfriend was great at first, but how patient can one young guy be? At first, he never pressured me to have sex or made me feel bad about what I was going through. But I think the stress eventually got to him, too. He started making snide comments regarding my lack of interest and constantly made me feel bad that I was too scared to try being intimate. To make matters worse, the antibiotics I was on gave me chronic yeast infections. So not only was he complaining about my lack of performance, but now commenting on the common side effect of my yeast infections. My confidence was gone.

Needless to say, the relationship ended and I moved on with my life. I had been accepted into a grad program and decided to change my area of concentration to sexuality education. I figured I should learn more about how my life had changed and how I can possibly prevent things like this for other women. I threw myself into my studies and loved every minute of it! I got involved in everything I could that related to sexual health. I had an awesome internship working at an amazing research institute helping with their student outreach program and I was also a student assistant to an incredible research group.

One night as we were entering data about women who worked for an in-home party plan, selling relationship enhancement products for one of our studies, I became intrigued with the information. We were trying to get an idea of who these women were, why they chose this career path and what they thought were the benefits of their job. I was enthralled reading about these women impacting other women on a regular basis. I wanted to be one of them—and that's how I found Pure Romance.

I am both relieved and proud to tell you that Colleen was able to recover, both physically and emotionally, from the trauma she experienced. And I share her story not to draw attention to her suffering or to the solace she found in Pure Romance, but as a cautionary tale: If only Colleen had had more education regarding her body and her sexuality, if she had received the information that most women need to supplement their natural lubrication with something as simple as a water-soluble lubricant, then she might have avoided her injury. If she had had the courage to tell her then-boyfriend that she didn't want to have sex, she might have avoided the entire episode. And if the physician had been more understanding, compassionate, and patient, he might have taken more time and care in treating Colleen.

As she herself said, "In hindsight, my biggest mistake was not listening to myself when I didn't want to have sex. I should have listened to my own cue and realized that it was okay to disappoint my boyfriend. In the hospital, I was a total puppet and wasn't the owner of my own body anymore. Since the accident, I have had very few orgasms. But I have been blessed to find a patient enough partner to deal with that. I know I will struggle with this the rest of my life and that childbirth will complicate the injury again. And even though my sexuality takes effort and energy, it's something I relish."

It is so important to take care of your sexual health, which often begins with paying attention and listening to what your body is telling you. Next, you should always find the best doctor possible, someone you trust, connect with, and who responds to your questions respectfully. If you are in the process of a move—whether you are relocating for a job or starting at a new college—take time to find a new doctor you are comfortable with and who will be able to offer you great resources. It is important to find a doctor who is going to be sensitive to your specific needs and guide you to any additional resources that may be helpful. In Colleen's case, it would have been a great relief to her to know that there were more options available to help her overcome the effects of her accident. She could have gone to couple's counseling to work through the issues in her relationship or seen a therapist for individual counseling to help her reconnect with her body in a positive way. Or a simple recommendation to use a lubricant during intercourse could have helped her in her attempts to try to be sexually active again with her boyfriend. Colleen had a wide variety of resources available to her to deal with her trauma and the changes to her body—someone just needed to open the door!

> In the National Health and Social Life Survey, 43 percent of American women had experienced sexual difficulties, and approximately 20 percent of women reported a lack of vaginal lubrication during sexual stimulation, with age, menopausal atrophy, vaginal dryness, and decreased sensation acting as contributing factors.*

When Sex Hurts

Colleen's story may seem exceptional, but many women tell me they experience pain or discomfort during sex. Pain during sex (dyspareunia) is common among women of all ages and may have several causes, some physiological, some more emotional. Sometimes it's related to hormonal changes that cause vaginal dryness; other times it's related to an undiagnosed infection; and still other times, it's related to nerve damage (as was the case with Colleen above). A number of other conditions can also impact a woman's ability to experience pleasure, inhibit her libido (some of these we touched upon in Chapter 2), and lessen her overall sexual

* Source: *JAMA*, Vol. 292, No. 14, 1999

functioning (usually related to her pelvis and her internal organs and tissues). Again, what's important to remember is that if you feel any discomfort either during sex or at other times, you should consult a physician or health care provider who knows about vulvo-vaginal pain. And these conditions can affect women in their teens, twenties, and up through their seventies. It's never too early or too late to begin paying attention to your sexual health.

Most problems with sexual health are labeled Female Sexual Disorders (FSDs), but I have a hard time with the limiting effect of labels. In my mind, the more we know precisely about how our bodies are working—or not working—the better able we are to get the help we need to correct those problems. As I mentioned in the previous chapter, the most common FSD is low libido that causes stress on you or in your relationship. But your sexuality is more than your libido and arousal. It includes your ability to orgasm, your ability to experience pleasure, incidence of pain, and degree of lubrication, and there are other sexual health conditions that also impact your sexual experience.

Do you remember the story of Amy, the widow who had gone so long without being sexually active that her vagina had literally atrophied (that is, prolapsed)? In another case, Mildred, a sixty-something woman told me that before she understood about the sexual health issues affecting her, she dreaded going to the doctor for her annual pap smear. "One year, I was so afraid, I called my daughter in tears. I didn't think I could get the courage to go to my appointment."

Why was she so afraid? Because she suffered such acute vaginismus (a tightening at the entry of the vagina) that even when a doctor tried to put a finger inside of her, she recoiled in pain. Her daughter, who happens to be a Pure Romance consultant, felt horrible that her mother had never shared this information with her. And it had been going on for years!

Thankfully, with the help of a vaginal dilator, Mildred's vaginismus gradually began to resolve, but not without demanding a lot of courage and patience on the part of Mildred.

Certain medical conditions, treatments, and surgeries can result in a narrowing of the vagina, decreased elasticity, muscle spasms, or genital pain. Pure Romance's vaginal dilator set includes six tapered devices to slowly stretch the vaginal walls, helping to make penetration or routine medical exams less painful. Vaginal dilators play an important role in a larger treatment plan recommended by your physician.

In another case, Sophia, a thirty-something woman, wrote in to me, describing "intense pain during intercourse." The official name for this kind of pain is dyspareunia (see page 77). When I asked her how long she had been experiencing this pain, she said, "Ever since I had surgery to have polyps [abnormal tissue growths] removed from my cervix." Any kind of surgery, but especially gynecological, can cause a change in vulvo-vaginal health. Intercourse may become painful when there is not enough moisture in the vagina or when the tissue lining becomes fragile. This also happens during menopause, when lower estrogen levels cause physical changes in a woman's sexual organs. For some women, taking hormone replacement therapy (HRT) can help. For others, the introduction of a vaginal moisturizer such as Fresh Start can help replenish the moisture lost in the tissue. This should be used in conjunction with your water-based lubricant.

Here is an overview of the most common causes of sexual pain, discomfort, or a lack of sensation during sex:

♡ **Vaginismus** refers to involuntary spasms of the muscles at the entry into the vagina. For some women, the spasms are so severe they cannot insert a finger or a tampon, never mind a penis.

♡ **Vulvar vestibulitis** refers to abnormal sensation at the entrance of the vulva (see the illustration in Chapter 2). Some women complain of tenderness, stinging, burning, urinary frequency, and pain in and around the area. There are many causes for vestibulitis, including insufficient hydration or lubrication, emotional stress, and shifts in hormones (i.e., a dramatic decrease in estrogen which promotes elasticity and lubrication).

♡ **Vulvodynia** is a condition that develops from vulvar vestibulitis, and refers to chronic pain and discomfort of the vulva area. Some types of vulvodynia are caused by infections such as candida (yeast), chronic vaginitis, and some herpes. Other forms of vulvodynia closely resemble vulvar vestibulitis, and cause burning, throbbing, itching, and stinging of the outer lips of the vagina. There is no one single cause. Some doctors believe vulva pain can be a result of skin problems, genetic factors, muscle spasms in the pelvis, allergies, and nerve damage to the vulva.

♡ **Dyspareunia** refers to pain during sex, specifically intercourse. Often a result of vulvar vestibulitis, dyspareunia is very common and is generally experienced either with initial penetration or more deeply, with thrusting during intercourse. Again, this pain rarely has a single cause, but is often a result of multiple factors, including vaginal infections or STDs; hormonal problems; vaginal abrasions, scars, or nerve damage (sometimes caused by trauma, abuse, or rough sex); too much or too little hygiene; insufficient vaginal lubrication; or vaginismus.

♡ **Chronic Pelvic Pain or Pelvic Inflammatory Disease (PID)** is marked by chronic pain with one of the organs in the pelvic area, including the uterus, ovaries, fallopian tubes, cervix, vagina, urinary tract, lower intestine, or rectum. It's often caused by a combination of vulvodynia, endometriosis, and uterine fibroids. Because its causes are multifactorial, treatment of PID needs to be handled by a knowledgeable and thorough physician or expert who can put together all the possible issues.

♡ **Anorgasmia** is the inability of women to achieve orgasm, even with adequate stimulation. Use of the word "inability" here should be qualified, however. Some women have never been able to achieve orgasm at any point in their life; other women have had orgasms on their own, but not with another person; and still other women have experienced orgasms in the past but can no longer experience a climax.

Often ob-gyn physicians are unfamiliar with these conditions. Some women have found the most effective diagnosis and treatment from dermatologists, interestingly enough, who may be more knowledgeable about the health of all the body's tissues. The best diagnosis and treatment is often found with physicians who specialize in vulvo-vaginal health. And know that many of these conditions respond to therapy—you may just need to go the extra mile to find the best help possible. (Please see the Resources section for further information.)

Intimacy Issue #3—Why Can't I Orgasm?
A Case of Sexual Dysfunction

Like many sexual dysfunctions, diagnosis of anorgasmia is somewhat subjective and depends a great deal upon the thoughts, emotions, and desires of the individual experiencing it. Some women may never achieve orgasm through intercourse with their partner and yet live active, fully satisfying sex lives by achieving orgasm in other ways, such as her partner manually stimulating her clitoris. Other women may be able to achieve orgasm through manual stimulation, yet still feel depressed, inadequate, and unfulfilled because they can not reach orgasm during intercourse. Studies show that up to 40 percent of adult American women have problems achieving orgasms.

Contributing factors include lack of sexual education,

strong religious upbringing, lack of strength in the woman's pubococcygeus (PC) muscle, past sexual abuse, impotence or early ejaculation in the male partner, and high levels of anxiety associated with sex. Although some of these explanations have shown a correlation with anorgasmic women, no one factor has been shown to significantly contribute to the problem any more than another.

Counseling for anorgasmic women will most likely focus on three areas. First, women are usually encouraged to attend sex therapy with their primary sexual partner. There are several reasons for this, but the principal one is that anorgasmia, like many sexual dysfunctions, cannot be seen solely as the woman's problem—many relationship variables can affect the symptom and, therefore, need to be treated in couples' therapy. Women are also taught to do kegel exercises (see page 104), and directed to masturbate to treat their orgasm problem. As you saw in Chapter 2, I am a big proponent of self-exploration and women learning how to bring themselves to orgasm. But please remember: inability to orgasm is a complex problem and you should uncover all the possible reasons and potential causes before you give up trying.

ASK PATTY:
BABY BLUES

Dear Patty,

I am a new mom; my beautiful baby girl has just turned five months old. I've heard women complain

before that after having a baby their sex drive
suffers. I always assumed it was a result of all the
new added pressures and chaos, understandably so.
I thought I would just have to make sure I put an
extra added effort into our intimate relationship to
keep it as strong as it has always been. Since I have
had the baby it hasn't just been the mental and
emotional restraints, it is also physical. I don't seem
to be able to get as aroused as I used to. Even
during sex, there doesn't seem to be as intense a
feeling as there was before. I am certainly not a
doctor, so I was curious as to whether nerves could
be damaged during the vaginal delivery? There are
also times when he hits a certain way during sex that
is extremely painful. This never was an issue before.
Now it is hard for him to relax during sex because
he's scared he's going to hurt me.

I have a very hardworking, attentive, wonderful
husband! I want to do anything possible to make
sure that we both enjoy a healthy, pleasurable
intimate relationship. Having a great intimate
relationship with my husband has always kept us
playful and given us a break from the day-to-day
insanity. Now it seems like it is more of an "issue" to
add to the pile of all of the other daily "issues" we
face. I desperately want to regain the intimacy and
playfulness that we had before and also have the
knowledge to help women in the same situation.

I apologize this was so long, I sincerely appreciate your help!

After Baby Blues

Dear After Baby Blues,

Welcome to the wonderful world of motherhood. Only a mother knows the unbelievable challenges mothers experience! But keep in mind that most of the time, intimacy returns and sex can get even better than it was before giving birth to your baby. You just need motivation and a few helpful hints from someone who has been there. Experts estimate that it takes two years for your body to fully recover from pregnancy and childbirth, and I think it is important to add the pure exhaustion of the first year of parenthood. Your body is absolutely experiencing changes in blood flow, as well as changes in your nerve sensations after pregnancy and childbirth. It is really common for women to feel less sensitive and have a harder time with arousal following childbirth. Changing body hormone concentrations also affect your sex drive and sensitivity level. All of these components together can have a huge impact on your physical and emotional capabilities to be intimate!

An important and easy step to take to regaining your intimate life is to maintain your vaginal health. Doing regular kegel exercises, or pelvic exercises, as well as paying attention to your post-baby body can help you adjust to the changes your body experiences after childbirth. What you are going through is normal, but know that you still need to rediscover your body by experimenting with new foreplay patterns, new positions, and new techniques. It is even possible for a woman's cervix to change position due to childbirth. Again, this is normal, but can be responsible for sharp, painful sensations if it is located at the back or top of your vagina. If this is so, try using more lubricant (you should always use a water-based lubricant during intercourse following childbirth). If you are still experiencing pain during penetration, try using the Super Stretch (see page 200) during intercourse until your body has healed properly. This allows you to enjoy only the amount of penetration that is comfortable for you and the Super Stretch will provide him with the full sensation he needs for stimulation.

I would also recommend some extended foreplay and to take it slow! When you are tired and extremely sensitive, additional foreplay and extra lubrication will enhance your level of comfort while your most sensitive areas are healing. Remember, the best gift to your child is a set of parents who still enjoy being husband and wife.

Truly,
Patty

Your sexual health is an important part of the overall health of your body. The more attuned to your body you are, the better able you will be to notice changes and attend to them quickly. I hope you refer to this book and its resources, as well as our website (www.pureromance.com) for any or all questions related to sexual health issues. And remember, the first step is a desire to learn.

I truly believe that no matter how old you are, you must take care of your sexual health. Though I am not a physician, as I mentioned earlier, I am convinced that women across this country have very little access to accurate, reliable information when it comes to their sexual functioning. I have heard and received far too many questions about pain during sex, sexually transmitted infections (STIs), birth control, the impact of medications, and the long-term effect of trauma on a woman's sexuality. It's crucial for women to know when something is not working right so that they can get the help they need and enjoy their sexuality throughout their lives. After all, don't we want to improve educational resources so that our daughters, nieces, and granddaughters will grow up to become empowered, confident women who know how to enjoy and protect their sexual health? So as you read this chapter and begin to consider your own sexual issues, know that I applaud you for taking the responsibility to protect and assure your own health. Like my own, the first step of your journey is the desire to learn.

CHAPTER FOUR

Putting the "O" Back in Romance

THE MIGHTY "O" has long been mythologized, feared, and considered elusive by many. I'd like to say two things: first, if there's a will, there's a way, and I am here to show you the many ways you can learn how to orgasm; and second, learning how to orgasm is a process. It's not an achievement, a goal, or a criterion for sexual pleasure or having great sex. So many women (and men!) put so much pressure on themselves to have an orgasm—and hindering themselves in the process not only by trying too hard but also by approaching the topic with an attitude that is goal-oriented rather than process-oriented. So know this: most women are able to orgasm once they relax, learn how their bodies respond to stimulation, and release into the sensation enough to become aroused.

As with everything related to sex, orgasms are as much an emotional skill as a physical skill. Specifically, you have to be relaxed enough to pay attention to how your body is feeling. Being able to keep this focus on just your sensual experience is often very difficult for women, who are so used to taking care of others or worrying about how their partner is feeling or doing that they have trouble shifting into "me mode."

Another big factor to keep in mind is that orgasms come in all shapes and sizes. There is no one way to have an orgasm, and there is no one place from where an orgasm emanates. For instance, some women experience a clitoral orgasm from direct and intense stimulation of their clitoris, but experience the actual peak of sensation way back in their vaginal walls. Other women prefer gentle, soft stimulation of the clitoris and then experience a small but intense pulsing that stems from the center of the clitoris. Still other women prefer gentle stimulation of the g-spot during intercourse or with a nonvibrating toy. How you achieve an orgasm is entirely personal and unique to what feels good to you. Just as no two snowflakes are alike, every orgasm is different.

Intimacy Issue #4—"I've never had an orgasm."

Many women are not sure whether they have ever experienced an orgasm. But most of the time, women can learn to have an orgasm—whether through manual or oral stimulation of the clitoris, through g-spot stimulation, or vaginally through intercourse. There are so many ways to explore your body, I hesitate even to label orgasms into "types"! Having an orgasm is a physical as well as a mental and emotional event. Women who have not yet learned to bring themselves to orgasm need to work on all of these areas before they are successful. Physically, as long as you have not had a pelvic injury or major pelvic surgery, you should be healthy enough to have an orgasm. Mentally, you need to make sure you are not harboring any lingering negative associations about sex that may be blocking you—perhaps you want to go back to the questionnaire in Chapter 1. And finally, emotionally, are you still suffering from the pain of a past breakup or divorce? Do you have a healthy body image? Have you experienced any situations that may have hurt you emotionally? Again, an orgasm is as much a mental and emotional experience as it is physical.

Most women learn to orgasm first from direct clitoral stimulation. Remember, the more pressure you put on yourself to do it, the more difficult this can become. Try some relaxation exercises or a nice, hot bath. Watch a sexy movie, read a romance novel, look at some erotica, or try whatever gives you a sexy sensation.

When you are feeling ready to take this a step further, I suggest using a nice lubricant to massage yourself, including all of your erogenous zones. Try rubbing your nipples, abdomen, and all parts of your vulva to provide added stimulation. Pay attention to the parts that feel the best. You can use a vibrating toy, such as Silver Bullet or Waterproof Power Bullet if you would like to have a little more control over your level of stimulation. Because the bullet delivers a more intense level of stimulation, some women find it easier to use when learning how to reach orgasm. Take your time. Too many times women say they give up after five or ten minutes because that is what they are used to seeing on TV. And remember, it is normal for a woman to enjoy twenty-five to forty-five minutes of foreplay before reaching orgasm. Enjoy the journey! Learn how your body likes to be touched and then the orgasm will happen naturally. It is important to not force it and just revel in the pleasurable sensations you are experiencing!

What Is an Orgasm?

Do you remember the graph I shared with you in Chapter 2, detailing the five stages of arousal? The first stage is a desire for sex, followed by the physical sensation of arousal; then women move into a general building of excitement, followed by a "plateau," which sometimes culminates in an orgasm. With arousal, women experience an increase in lubrication and a widening and lifting of the vagina (in some women, their vagina balloons), in order to make way for the penis. Of course, this arousal can happen without the presence of a penis.

From the strictly physiological point of view, an orgasm is the contraction of the upper third of the vagina and the uterus every eight-tenths of a second. Some women describe this sensation as a "quickening." Others say an orgasm feels "as if my heart is about to explode." Some describe it as their eyes rolling back in their head, toes curling, and their bodies shaking; some women have described it as an experience of their heart pounding and being out of breath. Other women say they "feel like they're in another world" or having an "out of body experience" or "a total loss of control."

Types of Orgasms

In general, there are three major types of orgasms: Clitoral, vaginal, and g-spot. Women can also experience orgasms in different places around their body, including their breasts, nipples, and anus (especially during anal sex), but I am going to focus on the more common ones.

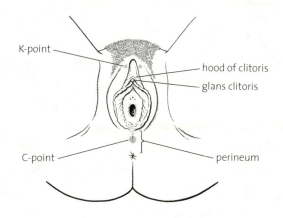

CLITORAL

Some women affectionately refer to the clitoris as "the little man in the boat," or their "precious little flower." But some women really don't even know where it is. So before reading anything more, why don't you grab a hand mirror and make sure you can locate your clitoris, then you'll be in a much better position to know how to make yourself orgasm. And keep in mind that this tiny area is packed with nerve endings (eight thousand plus) that have no function other than to bring you pleasure.

The clitoral orgasm is the most common and, for some women, the strongest orgasm. Most women need some form of clitoral stimulation to orgasm. A clitoral orgasm occurs when the clitoris is stimulated to peak excitement. Typically, the sensation starts within the clitoral area and may radiate out from there. The nerve system involved uses the pudendal nerve system (the set of nerves that connect the pelvic area to the genitals), which is made up of highly sensitive nerve fibers. The clitoris glans (what we usually call the bud) is the only visible part of a woman's clitoris, yet it's been found that the clitoris is actually ten times larger than previously thought, extending back into the vaginal walls. In general women experience clitoral orgasms from manual touching, oral stimulation, vibrators, and other enhancers. But because the "legs" of the clitoris (the highly sensitive nerve fibers) extend way inside, women can experience a clitoral orgasm either internally or externally. There are certain intercourse positions that are especially good for clitoral stimulation, whether or not you reach orgasm; these include female superior, side by side, or standing (with the male partner sitting, on a chair for example).

G-SPOT

The g-spot was named in honor of the German physician Ernst Grafenberg, who first noted its existence, and was made famous by Dr. Beverly Whipple. Approximately the size of a dime, the g-spot is located about two-thirds the length of your middle finger inside the vaginal entrance, on the "tummy" side of the front vaginal wall. Because of its position, many women have trouble locating their g-spot. And Dr. Beverly Whipple points out that the "g-spot is not in the vaginal wall, but felt through it," and therefore requires more direct and firm pressure to simulate it. With one or two fingers, reach inside your vagina about two or three inches, positioning your fingers upward toward the top side of the vaginal wall until you feel a slightly ruffled area of tissue. Using a "come hither motion," gently stroke this area. As the area becomes callous in texture and grows both more puffy and bigger in size, keep stroking steadily. Remember, it takes a lot of stimulation to find the g-spot, which is why a g-spot vibrator works so well in this area.

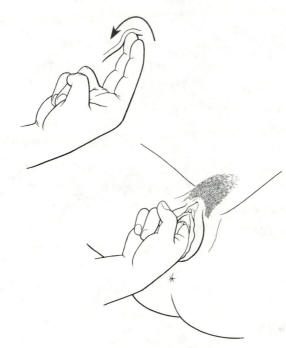

About My G-Spot . . .

Hi Patty,

First, I want to thank you for your wonderful products! Second, I want to thank you even more for a place where I can ask really sensitive questions. I would like to know if clitoral stimulation is needed for a g-spot orgasm. The reason I ask is that a clitoral orgasm is achieved very easily for me, but it seems to be a prelude to something bigger and better. I have never experienced a g-spot orgasm. Is it the same thing, but achieved by stimulating a different place? Or is it a new experience? Having my clitoris stimulated too much during sex seems to be kind of distracting and takes away from a different kind of pleasure. My husband (who actually taught me how to achieve clitoral orgasm by myself) laments that I don't have one during sex except for sometimes when he is concentrating on the outside of me rather than the inside. I am thinking about purchasing the G-Wiz, and I guess I am hoping to experience something a little different.

Again, thanks for providing a place where I can ask this.

Anonymous

Dear Anonymous,

Thank you for bringing the g-spot out into the open. It sounds like you and your husband have a great relationship and are continuing to keep a fabulous intimate connection.

Let me start at the beginning. The g-spot is a cluster of sensitive, spongy tissue that surrounds your urethra, which is the tube that carries urine from your bladder out of your body. The g-spot tissue swells as you get aroused, much like your clitoris or the lips of your vagina. When you are aroused, you will find the sensitive tissue about two or three inches inside your vagina, toward your abdomen. The g-spot isn't actually in your vagina, but you can stimulate it from the vagina. You have to apply some pressure to press through the front muscular wall of your vagina to feel the full effects of g-spot stimulation. From the inside, aim your pressure toward your natural pubic hairline on the outside. The g-spot is about the size of a quarter when you are really aroused.

Most women concur that the g-spot becomes more sensitive after you are really aroused. You can do this through clitoral stimulation and orgasm or by lots of foreplay. Since you have experienced and enjoy clitoral stimulation, I would recommend having one or more clitoral orgasms before you begin stimulating the g-spot area. You may want to continue to stimulate the clitoris as you begin to stimulate the front wall of your vagina.

It may take a couple of tries to locate and stimulate your g-spot. Be patient with your body. The G-Wiz will be a great way to help you explore g-spot stimulation. Be sure to pair the toy with a lubricant for maximum benefit.

Good luck and happy exploring!

Truly,
Patty

Vaginal Orgasm

A vaginal orgasm tends to be deeper and more diffuse in sensation than the "spot-on" nature of a clitoral orgasm. Women with very toned and strong PC muscles are more likely to experience this type of sexual sensation, usually from continual squeezing of the penis during penetration. (This is what you are strengthening when you are doing a kegel exercise.)

In addition, some women need clitoral stimulation during penetration in order to reach a vaginal orgasm. Positions that enable strong vaginal wall stimulation are male superior, rear entry, and for women with extraordinarily strong PC muscles, female superior. Most women require manual stimulation of the g-spot to reach an orgasm, while some women can position their partner in such a way as to create friction and stroking with his penis during penetration and gentle thrusting. But remember, most women require clitoral stimulation during sex to even have an orgasm. Some women can have a g-spot orgasm from rear entry or doggie style if the man can precisely stimulate the g-spot with his penis. So keep in mind that you can adjust your position. As one woman described, "it's not exactly like doggie; it's kind of doggie off to the side." In other words, if you would like your partner to stimulate your g-spot during intercourse, be aware enough to make the shifts in position that you need. (You will find more information about which positions enable which types of orgasms in Chapter 9.)

Female Ejaculation

Many women are confused about, bothered by, or afraid of female ejaculation. Let me first explain what it is. Research has now documented that some women release a fluid from the urethra during sex, but this fluid is not urine. Some researchers imply that female ejaculation may be somewhat analogous to male ejaculation! Some women are surprised when they ejaculate. As Kris said, "My husband and I were making love and had a longer than average foreplay—he'd given me oral sex and vice versa and then we really took a long time during intercourse. When we both finally reached orgasm, I let out this burst of fluid. I think it was because I was so in tune with my body and what was happening and every part of me was excited." Kris loved the feeling and says, "Now I try to ejaculate—I usually have to be on top and have to focus a lot—but I love the sense of power it gives me, and my husband is totally into it!"

Of course, female ejaculation is certainly not a requirement for an orgasm (whether clitoral, vaginal, or g-spot). Let your body direct you—the more in tune you are with how you are responding to sensation, the more pleasure you will experience.

ASK PATTY:
Failing at the G-Spot

Dear Patty,

I'd like some information on g-spot orgasms. My husband and I found the g-spot many years ago and it's a great way to "get me warmed up." My clitoris is hypersensitive for a few days after my period so I don't like having it stimulated and will try for a g-spot orgasm instead. Unfortunately this usually makes me feel as if I'm going to urinate. In fact, the more I'm enjoying myself, the worse it gets. So of course I tense up, which ruins the orgasm.

At a Pure Romance party I held at my house, my consultant talked about g-spot orgasms and mentioned that most women tense up because they think they're going to urinate. She told us to just relax and enjoy the sensation and it should pass.

So, the next time I did relax and . . . guess what?

After I experienced an intense orgasm I also experienced a huge puddle on the bed. My husband had to get a paper towel for his hand; I was mortified and ended up cleaning up with the same stuff I use for the puppy. I had emptied my bladder before we started, so I thought everything would be fine. Obviously I'm doing something wrong. Can you help?

Sincerely,
Failing at the G-Spot

Dear Failing at the G-Spot,

You are not failing at all! You have just experienced a female ejaculation! Congratulations! Men are not the only ones that are capable of ejaculating. Women are also completely capable of ejaculating with intense stimulation and sometimes deep g-spot stimulation.

Your Pure Romance consultant was right to tell you that you are not urinating when you are aroused, even though it may feel as if you do. When you experience an intense orgasm, sometimes from a g-spot orgasm, it causes a muscle contraction that forces a watery, lubricating fluid out of your urethra. Although it may feel like you just wet the bed, it is not urine! It does leave your body through the same tube, but it is a completely different fluid.

Please do not be embarrassed! Female ejaculate is completely normal and does not have an odor or leave a stain. You may need to use a towel or change the sheets after experiencing such an intense orgasm, but it usually feels so good, you don't care. Only about 10 to 20 percent of women know they

ejaculate, so consider yourself among an elite club of
satisfied women! I hope you try it again!

> Truly,
>
> Patty

What Can Inhibit Orgasm

As mentioned in the previous chapter, many conditions can contribute to difficulty having an orgasm. Some women who have
never experienced an orgasm are said to be "anorgasmic," or suffer
from "anorgasmia." However, I like to think that unless they have
experienced severe physiological trauma to the nerve endings of
their clitoris, vulva, or vagina, most women can develop sensation
that can lead to an orgasm or some sexual pleasure. That said,
there are lifestyle habits that you need to avoid if you want to increase your chances of having an orgasm or make the ones you are
experiencing more enjoyable or pleasurable. And it's also true that
some women have such intense, long-standing emotional issues
tied to trauma that they can never let go enough to experience an
orgasm. So even if they stay away from any of these orgasm "inter-
rupters," they might still not be able to orgasm.

♡ **High fatty or high starch diet.** A diet that is high
in fat contributes to hypertension (high blood pressure), high cholesterol, and inflammation. Basi-
cally, all these precursors to heart disease also work
against orgasms. Especially true for men (who need
a lot of healthy blood flow to support an erection),
this is also true for women whose bodies rely on
strong circulation as a way of staying "orgasmically

fit" and able to create sensation. If you have diabetes or are significantly overweight you will also have a decreased capacity for orgasm.

♡ **Smoking.** Smoking is bad not only for your lungs, but for your overall health. And when you smoke, you stress your circulatory system, which is a necessary component to healthy sexuality, especially orgasms.

♡ **Stress.** As discussed earlier, any kind of stress— emotional, mental, or physical—can truly dampen your ability to orgasm.

♡ **Sleep.** We are a sleep deprived nation. We stay up late, watch too much television, take a lot of stimulants, and our sex lives suffer. The more regular sleep patterns you have, the better your overall health . . . and the stronger and more reliable your orgasms.

♡ **Antidepressants.** Medicines that boost (or balance) serotonin have been shown to lessen both libido and the ability to orgasm. As mentioned, only one, Wellbutrin, does not raise serotonin and has actually been tied to an increase in orgasmic response. Make sure to talk to your health care provider to find the right antidepressants for you. They can help you find a medication with appropriate side effects for your sexual health.

♡ **Trauma to the clitoris or vulva.** Any kind of nerve damage to the clitoris, vulva, or vagina can impair your ability to experience sexual sensation, including an orgasm. However, do not despair. As you will see in Chapter 9, Moving Beyond Missionary, there are other ways to experiment sexually and discover new routes to sexual and sensual pleasure.

♡ **Weak PC muscles.** Renowned sex researcher and author Dr. Beverly Whipple has shown that strong PC muscle tone is directly related to vaginal orgasmic ability. So no matter how little strength you may have in this area, you can—and should—do something about it! (See more info on kegels and strengthening your PC muscles below.)

ASK—PATTY:
Looking for the Big O

Dear Patty,

I have been with my boyfriend for seven years; we have only been sexually active for three years. In all this time I have not had an orgasm. Is there something wrong with me? I really appreciate your help, as I don't know who else to ask!

Sincerely,
Looking for the Big O

Dear Looking for the Big O,

I am always excited when women write me for tips on having their first orgasm. Orgasms are a healthy part of anyone's life, providing a whole list of benefits, including stress reduction, mental clarity, decreased depression, and boosted self-esteem. Having an orgasm is a skill not unlike riding a bike. The difference is someone usually teaches you how to ride a bike!

The first thing that I recommend is that you take the time to explore your own body. Spend some time alone and find the areas that bring you pleasurable sensations, as well as learn which areas bring you to orgasm when stimulated. Once you have a greater understanding of your "hot spots" you can share what you learned with your boyfriend. Orgasm is as much mental as it is a physical response and we have found that sometimes women pressure themselves too much to reach orgasm in the presence of their partners. I promise that you will benefit tremendously by figuring things out on your own and then integrating what you've learned when you are with your boyfriend.

Choose a time when you are relaxed, put on some music, light a few candles, and turn off the phone. Think about when you feel most aroused and anything else you find sexy that may help get you in the mood. Read a sexy novel, watch a movie that turns you on and pay attention to the parts of the story that give you the most pleasure. Next get a nice water-based lubricant, sit in front of a big mirror, and take some time to fully explore your genitals. If you have never taken a good look at your genitals, you may benefit from this experience. As you explore, pay attention to which parts feel the most sensitive. Most women achieve orgasm by stimulating the clitoris (on the outside) rather than inside the vagina.

While you are exploring, I recommend applying a pea-sized amount of an arousal cream to your clitoris. A heightener will give you a tingly feeling and enhance your sexual response and is great for first-time users. It is not necessary to use a vibrator, but some women find it helpful as you learn how your body likes to be touched in order to reach orgasm. A bullet is a small, hand-held vibrating toy that provides a higher level of stimulation. Think of the bullet as training wheels. You will not always want or need to use it, but right now, it will help guide you. Orgasms are intense, sometimes overwhelming feelings. You may feel like you are losing control and that is normal. Play with the bullet, move it around to all of the sensitive spots that you found earlier. When it feels good, hold it there.

As you get more aroused and closer to orgasm, you will feel your breathing increase and you heart beat faster. As you experience increasing feelings in your genitals, relax and let yourself go. Don't make this too much like a science experiment and don't think so much that you psych yourself out as you get close. Think sexy thoughts. Most women need about twenty-five to forty-five minutes of foreplay to reach orgasm, but you may desire or require even more as you are learning. It may take a couple of tries as you get used to this new experience, but I know you can do it. Good luck! Great things are just around the corner!

Truly,
Patty

What You Can Do
to Strengthen Your Orgasm

If you are ready, willing, and open to exploring your body, there are ways to strengthen your body and hone your mind-set to enjoy better orgasms.

The Right Attitude

♡ Have fun! If you take yourself too seriously, or are trying too hard to "get there," you will simply get in your own way. The chemistry of orgasm is delicate and one of its most crucial aspects is staying loose—in your body and your head. When you approach sex in general and orgasms specifically as a time for you and your partner to have fun or for you to have fun on your own, you increase the odds for reaching an orgasm.

♡ Take your time! Again, orgasms stem from a mind-body-heart connection, which means you need to give yourself enough time and space to relax and let your body lead you. If you're with a partner, then encourage him (or her) to be patient, and be patient with yourself as well.

♡ Be selfish. If you want to orgasm, you need to be able to tune out and focus only on your body's sensation. Why do you think so many women close their eyes just before they climax? Because this enables them to concentrate and pay extra-close attention to each building second toward orgasm. Being selfish doesn't mean you don't care about your partner or his pleasure; it simply means that you know how to focus on your own.

A Better Body for Sex

♡ Strengthen your PC muscles. There is no doubt about it, the stronger and more toned your PC muscles, the more able you are to orgasm, and the richer and deeper the experience. Our doctors should be telling us to do our kegels from early on. And now it's a lot easier with such tricks as Ben Wa balls and other "kegelcisors"—these tools are like lifting weights with your vagina!

Practice, Practice, Practice

♡ Pay attention. When you take time to get to know your body, you are better able to cue into how it is responding, which in turn will help you focus on the mounting tension that leads to orgasm.

♡ Practice with a vibrator or bullet. These handy items are the fastest, most effective way for a woman to learn how to orgasm through clitoral stimulation. They vary in speed, intensity, and size, so a woman—on her own terms—can discover her own route to pleasure.

Remember, orgasms are all about being process oriented rather than goal oriented. The more you take your time, get comfortable, and practice by yourself or with a partner who is supportive, loving, and cued into you and your body, the better your chances for putting the "O" back in your love life or discovering it on your own for the very first time.

How to Do a Kegel

1. Lie down on your bed, the floor, or a mat with your knees bent and your feet on the floor.
2. Find the muscles inside your vagina by squeezing them as if to stop the flow of urine.
3. As you squeeze, count to five and then release.
4. Repeat in groups of ten, building toward twenty-five, then fifty.

Once you become familiar with how to isolate your PC muscle, you can do your kegels virtually anywhere—in your car or at your desk—whenever or wherever you remember to do them. You can also strengthen these muscles using Ben Wa balls, small weights that act as resistance trainers. Ideally, women should do kegels every day to strengthen and tone this band of muscle. Not only do kegels improve the overall health of your pelvis, especially after childbirth and as you age, but you will also notice that it is easier for you to become physically aroused and you might even experience more intense clitoral and vaginal orgasms. In fact, research has shown that kegel exercises improve sexual arousal in women!

Of course, excellent PC muscle tone also has the added benefit of giving a woman a tighter vagina, something both women and their partners can appreciate. Excellent PC muscle tone also indirectly helps clitoral orgasms by improving circulation and also stimulating the further end of the clitoris. So doing kegels—with or without a resistance device—will indeed make clitoral orgasms more sharp and intense.

A Word About Multiple and Simultaneous Orgasms

The biggest factor in any kind of orgasm, but especially if you and your partner want to try to orgasm together, is your mutual ability to pay attention to your own body and your partner's—and this means becoming finely tuned in to timing. Over 60 percent of women require some sort of clitoral stimulation in order to orgasm. In order to create the sensation and the timing for a couple to climax together, either a woman needs to be touching herself, her partner needs to touch her or be in a position that enables clitoral stimulation, or they need to use a bedroom accessory such as a Jelly Tool Belt (see page 198 for an illustration of this adaptable toy, as well as more info on others!).

Women who are able to orgasm from g-spot stimulation, or from another kind of vaginal orgasm, may be able to learn precise control of their PC muscles in order to cue into their partner's sensations to orgasm simultaneously. Some sex experts also recommend the coital alignment technique (CAT), which involves the man being able to position himself on top of the woman in such a way that he is deeply inside of her, while maintaining constant motion and contact with the woman's clitoris. The direct contact between the base of his penis and her clitoris is what stimulates her clitoris while he is approaching orgasm. (For more information see Chapter 9.)

When it comes to multiple orgasms, it is really about the individual. Some women are able to orgasm only once during a single encounter, and other women have multiple or varied orgasms within a single lovemaking session. Again, it's a waste of time and energy to worry about this—having multiple orgasms doesn't necessarily make you a *better* lover; it just means you can have more orgasms during sex.

Remember, as you begin to implement some of this advice into your love life, one of the most important things to keep in mind is that orgasms change. Just as your body changes day to day, month to month, and year to year, so too does your style of orgasm. Some women have also told me that their orgasms change with each new partner. As Danielle, forty-six, said, "With my ex-husband, my main kind of orgasm was a deep, vaginal orgasm. He was never that into even trying to touch my clitoris or finding my g-spot. Now with my partner of ten years, I've expanded my repertoire, so to speak. He is so much more adventuresome and attentive, and I've discovered that I can orgasm from g-spot stimulation and with oral stimulation of my clitoris—something I was never relaxed enough to do with my ex."

So ladies, never limit yourselves—you never know what kind or orgasm may be waiting for you around that corner!

PART TWO

Turning to Your
Relationship

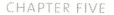

CHAPTER FIVE

Pillow Talk

Learning How to Stay Close

T MAY SOUND like a tired cliché—one we've all heard—but it remains true and bears repeating that if couples do not keep the channels of communication open, their relationship will wither away. In all my years helping women and men resuscitate their sex lives, most of my time is spent helping them relearn how to communicate with each other. Did you know that lack of communication is the number-one reason couples cite for why they are unhappy in their relationship or why their marriage ended in divorce? Who wants to be a part of that statistic?

Take Natalie and John, who were married for twenty years after being high school sweethearts. Needless to say, being together for over twenty years is a challenge for any couple—even the most committed! So though Natalie and John loved each other, they were also in a serious rut. They had faced several daunting challenges during their time together, including their youngest daughter's disability and John's getting laid off from his job at a textile company. Nonetheless, they had weathered through, always turning to each other for love and comfort. On the surface, they seemed like the ideal couple, still determined to work on their marriage after more than two decades.

But when I met Natalie, she confessed that she felt really distant from John. She found herself not sharing the details of her day with him, and not even working up the energy to try to anymore. Most nights they fell asleep after watching a string of television programs, and neither of them seemed much in the mood for sex—except maybe once a month when John would make a move and Natalie would respond, more out of guilt than interest.

When I asked Natalie point-blank what was going on, she said, "We have nothing to say to each other anymore."

"But you still love each other, right?"

Yes, she nodded.

"And you want to make this marriage last, right?"

Again, she nodded.

"And you want the years to pass pleasurably, with the two of you feeling connected, right?"

Right.

I explained that just as you put in the time and effort to maintain your car, home, or lawn to ensure that it will last into the future, your relationship also requires regular and consistent maintenance—and the key to this tune-up is being *willing* to communicate.

It's true: most of the work of relationships happens via communication. There has to be a mutual commitment to talking things out, and a strict policy of staying in touch verbally. There's no doubt that when couples stay connected, when they know each other's thoughts and feelings (well, most of them anyway!), they keep trust in place. That emotional and psychological bond is crucial to keeping the love alive. So that even in times of stress, whatever its source, couples can tap into a reservoir of emotional stability and intimacy and pump energy back into their relationship.

Let's face it: Natalie and John's story is a familiar one to many of us. Busy taking care of kids at home and careers at the office, many couples simply run out of steam before finding the time and space to tend to their relationship on a regular basis. Even couples who love each other, who are committed, and who want their relationship to be lively and sexy, and full of affection and closeness, still find themselves feeling out of sync and out of practice—or as Natalie said, "With nothing to say to each other anymore." And, like Natalie and John, a lack of communication *outside* the bedroom often means there's not much going on *inside* the bedroom.

The road back to a love connection might seem impossibly long and difficult. But it's not! Reconnecting with your partner takes work, but trust me, the process can be fun and gratifying—both physically and emotionally—and you will be rewarded with lasting, life-enhancing benefits to your sex life, your health, and your relationship as a whole.

When it comes to communicating with your partner about sex, here's one of the first steps: know thyself. I've spent the first part of this book helping you get in touch with your own desires, helping you learn to discover how your body works, how you respond to stimulation, and what gives you pleasure. You've become more aware of your sexual experiences over your lifetime, how those experiences have shaped you and, in turn, how you've changed. Now it's time to start sharing that wonderful new self-knowledge with your partner, and it's also time to start learning about your partner's desires. Believe me, whether you're a young couple just starting out or a long-married duo, there's a lot you can learn about each other that will surprise and delight you, while bringing you closer together.

Knowledge really is power. Just as you can embrace the power of being a woman by taking responsibility for your own sexuality, you and your partner, by entering into a loving, honest sexual conversation, can tap into a deep, powerful connection. This connection has all sorts of obvious benefits for your lovemaking, and it will also help to protect and sustain the health and well-being of your relationship at every level.

Back to Basics

Good communication is based on three key things: trust, acceptance, and openness. But before we even go into how to get better at communicating with your partner, you need to make sure both of you acknowledge and understand why communication is so important. Lasting, meaningful communication involves give and take on the part of both partners:

♡ Trusting and being trustworthy

♡ Being honest about your needs and accepting the needs of your partner

♡ Listening and sharing

Bringing this give-and-take into your bedroom will energize your sex life, which in turn will help you feel closer even when sex is the furthest thing from your minds.

The first step is to make a commitment to saying what is on your mind. How do you make a commitment to communicate? You remind yourself that if you stop talking, you stop relating, and then it's a domino effect, with all levels of communication breaking down along the way. But once the two of you acknowledge how important it is to stay close, you will be much more motivated to find a way to keep talking—through periods of stress, differences, or conflicts.

Trust

Healthy communication also requires that both of you feel safe and secure enough to share your thoughts and feelings, especially those that make you feel vulnerable or uneasy. This requires trust between partners, and trust can be weakened and eroded when you neglect your relationship. Not talking to your partner about how you feel, holding back anger and disappointment, avoiding conflict—these are all easy habits for couples to fall into, and they are all behaviors that undermine trust in a relationship. And just as avoidance and withholding can and will undermine trust, so will lashing out in anger, deliberately trying to hurt each other's feelings, and taking things out on each other. If your relationship has suffered from this kind of isolation and hurtfulness, you and your partner need to find ways to rebuild and shore up the bonds of trust between you. You need to get talking—and listening—again.

Reintroducing small, thoughtful gestures into your routine as a couple can help you start taking better care of your relationship, and it can help you *want* to talk to each other more. Here's a simple activity for you and your partner to try: Each of you takes a sheet of paper and makes a list of the small things the other person does regularly that make you feel loved. Write down everything you can think of, no gesture is too small or too simple. The list can include anything from holding your hand in the car to kissing you at the end of the day, from pouring you a cup of coffee in the morning to snuggling while you watch television at night. Once you've both made your lists, each of you adds three small gestures you wish your partner would do more often. These, too, can be anything—maybe you'd love your partner to read to you in the evenings, or bring you flowers once a week, or put on music and dance with you in the living room. Maybe he'd love you to scratch his back or pick up his favorite take-out meal for dinner and a movie at home. Once you've compiled your lists, it's time to share them. Swap lists, and over the next week, try to do one special thing from your partner's list every day. You don't have to discuss the lists, or what you plan to do. Just surprise each other with these simple, thoughtful gestures—and other sweet nothings that may not have made the lists—and you'll soon see how rewarding it is to both give and receive acts of tenderness and kindness.

You and your partner will build, or rebuild, trust when you share even the smallest moments together. Suddenly the conflicts seem smaller and it becomes easier to talk and listen to each other. (Soon, we'll work on taking this renewed trust and attention to one another's needs into the bedroom.)

Acceptance

As individuals, we all communicate differently. As a result, the very definition of "healthy communication" can take on a number of meanings, depending on the people involved. So how can we define such a subjective, individual concept? For some couples, good communication is being able to signal when they want to have a quickie; for others, good communication is simply saying, "I missed you today" or "I really love it when you rub my feet."

Still others show good communication skills when they are able to sit down and explain why they are angry or hurt or frustrated. Good communication is not a one-size-fits-all proposition: Creating healthy communication in your relationship is about identifying what sort of communication works for you and for your partner. If you are both inclined to talk things through, then great—you are probably also more comfortable having a good argument than some couples.

You and your partner may have similar communication styles, or you may be very different. Sometimes one person values restraint and calm, while the other needs to pour out his or her heart, even if things get heated. There is no single best way to communicate. The challenge for couples is to identify and accept whatever differences might exist in their communication styles, and then not allow those differences to prevent them from connecting with each other.

As women, we're often the ones to initiate communication. And you may just need to continue to be the one to initiate, even when it's tiresome or downright annoying that your partner seems to wait for you to take the driver's seat. I am not saying you should always let your partner off the hook or that he (or she) shouldn't take responsibility for beginning a conversation, but couples can waste a lot of time and energy staying silent in protest, when they might be having a more rewarding and fun relationship if they simply opened the door.

Openness

The more trust and acceptance are in place, the more naturally in tune you are with each other. Communication can then become less of a conscious effort and more something you do enjoyably and automatically. Once you're thinking about your partner and how to make him or her feel good and cared for, you will begin to share your hopes and your fears, and your thoughts about your future together. This emotional openness will grow because the trust is there, and because you know your partner is truly listening. In other words, the more you get in the habit of sharing your thoughts and feelings, the more you continue to pave the way to vital, real communication—the kind that weathers storms and is built to last.

ASK PATTY:
Waiting for Oral Pleasure

Hi Patty,

I have a boyfriend and I love him very much. The problem is that he does not know how to go down on me. He has tried before but has not been very successful. How can I tell him or show him how to do it, without making him feel bad? (I have not told him he is not very good at it.)

Attn, Waiting!

Dear Waiting,

It can be difficult to tell someone how to do something differently because it could hurt their feelings. However, this is not always the case. If your partner is interested in pleasing you, he may like the input and advice. Plus, having open lines of communication is an important part of any relationship. Offering your partner suggestions for how to perform oral favors may help strengthen the bond between you two. You could start the conversation with something like this: "I read in a magazine/book/ online about a new technique that I thought we could try. Do you want to hear it?" and then offer him suggestions for how to lick, touch, and tickle. You don't have to tell him that he's not very good; you can instead focus on how to make it better.

It is hard for me to give advice about how your boyfriend should perform oral favors because each person varies in how they like it. Think about what you enjoy and offer some suggestions during the act—"a little to the left" or "a little more pressure." You could also do something to show that he's doing it right (i.e., moaning or grabbing his head in delight). If you do this enough times, he will probably get the hint as to how to do it in the future.

You might want to read Sadie Allison's book *Tickle Your Fancy*. Although it is written for a female reader, is also the perfect book for men to learn more about what brings women pleasure. An easy way to get him to read it is to leave it in the bathroom. If you read it first, you could highlight parts that you are interested in trying. Or you could read the book and talk about it over dinner with him, suggesting that he read it too because it was so interesting. I hope this helps!

Truly,
Patty

Small Steps Mean Big Improvements

There are many ways to stay connected with your partner, and it's not all about sitting down and talking things through. The plans you make together, the activities you participate in as a couple, the ways you share in your daily and weekly routines, and the traditions you establish over time all help to strengthen your connection with your partner. But the bottom line is this: the point of communication is to strengthen your bond to each other. When that bond is maintained and cared for, then the communication will flow—in whatever style is most natural to you and your partner.

One of my favorite stories is about a couple I met in Naples, Florida. George and Lisette (their real names) have been together for twenty years, married for twelve. George is around thirty-seven and he and Lisette were high school sweethearts. As George said of himself, "I was the nerdy guy in high school but there was just something about Lisette—I just always adored her." On their very first date George took Lisette to a crab shack on the beach in their hometown. He was so nervous that he couldn't eat a thing. But after dinner, they took a walk on the beach to get to know each other. That night was a memorable, magical encounter.

Later, when they moved to Naples, one of the first things they did was search out a setting—a restaurant near a beach—that reminded them of their first date. And now each year on their anniversary, they re-create the magic of that first evening together: they order the same meal (though now George is able to eat his dinner) and afterward they take their beach walk. They make this night a priority in their lives, a time to check in on each other and rediscover who they are.

So you might not have a crab shack like George and Lisette, but you can shop around and create your own special tradition with your partner. Because anything worth having is worth working on. This annual tradition helps keep George and Lisette solidly grounded in the romance of their relationship, and this way of connecting is in itself a form of communication. So whether it's a crab shack in southern Florida or a fancy Italian restaurant, couples need to devise rituals and traditions to celebrate their relationship—it's what helps create your own special joint history.

One woman I know celebrates her anniversary by preparing a special dinner at home and then putting on her wedding dress so that she and her husband can relive the night they were married.

Think back to when you were dating. Did you have a favorite restaurant where you used to go for special occasions? Was there a special park or beach where you took walks together? Even something as simple as a song you both love can bring you back to times of happiness and excitement in your relationship. So jump in the car and head to that long-ago picnic spot, or pull out your old CD collection and see what happens!

If your old traditions no longer feel relevant or meaningful, do not despair. This just means you have the opportunity to create new ones. Finding ways to enjoy each other will come naturally if you allow yourselves to try new things on a whim. You probably think you know yourselves and each other through and through, but I believe everyone carries a little bit of mystery inside and it can be lots of fun discovering a new side to the person you thought you knew completely. Okay, you may be thinking. "I'm so busy, I don't have time to be that creative and spontaneous." Don't worry, it's all about small choices, which can add up to great rewards. Injecting a little spontaneity into your relationship doesn't have to take up a tremendous amount of time, nor does it require big changes or momentous decisions. It can be as simple as experimenting with a new recipe for dinner, catching an early movie on a weeknight when the kids are busy with their own activities, or deciding to spend an hour on a sunny afternoon working side-by-side in the garden. You might go the extra step and sign up for a cooking class or a ballroom dancing lesson, rent a tandem bicycle and go for a ride, or spend the night at a nearby inn and enjoy a night away from kids, pets, and household chores.

Date nights, whether they mark a special occasion like George and Lisette's, or are simple weekly outings for a leisurely meal and a glass of wine, are a great way to reintroduce romance into your relationship. And whatever your plans on date night, be sure to treat it like a real date! Put some thought into getting ready; consider wearing a flirty new dress or a sparkling piece of jewelry that you typically save for special events. Let yourself indulge in the pleasure of dressing up, and in the anticipation of meeting your sweetheart for a night out. No distractions, no interruptions. Just the two of you. These weekly rendezvous can reintroduce you to the funny, charming, passionate person you fell for in the first place.

ASK PATTY:
When Couples Stop Having Sex

Dear Patty,

I am worried about my sister. She and her husband have decided to stop having sex. They don't have any medical reasons; they just decided to stop.

I was wondering what you thought of this and if their relationship will suffer as a result. I am trying to support her decision but I am worried that this will hurt her in the long run.

Sincerely,
A Concerned Sister

Dear Concerned Sister,

Your sister is very lucky to have someone who is concerned about her happiness and well-being. From professional experience, we know there are physical and emotional ramifications for a couple experiencing a lack of intercourse. However, if a couple has made a mutual decision to stop engaging in intercourse but maintains a physically intimate relationship with massage, cuddling, holding hands, etc., as well as maintaining a healthy level of communication, the potential downsides to a relationship are greatly reduced. Physically, without regular release from intimate interaction when previously used to it, women will experience more sex dreams and men (if they are not masturbating) will experience nocturnal emissions (wet dreams).

We do know that physically, orgasms have many benefits to both men and women, including the release of endorphins, which are the body's natural good-feeling and pain-killing chemicals. Regular orgasms from sex also improve overall feelings of happiness and decrease feelings of depression. The release of oxytocin promotes feelings of attachment, which improves levels of commitment and boosts self-esteem.

Unfortunately, without regular sexual relations, a

couple often stops touching and communicating, which leads to a breakdown in the relationship. It is really important for your sister and her husband to truly understand why they've chosen to stop having sex. Men and women can use sex—or lack of sex—to manipulate or punish each other, which will only erode the relationship over time. It might be beneficial for couples to seek counseling if they view the cessation of sexual intercourse as a negative issue or if they are not completely in sync with the reasons for the decision. To find a certified therapist in your area, please visit www.aasect.org.

If, however, your sister and her husband made this decision together and are happy with it, then it is your responsibility to support her! Having sex is not the only way for a couple to be intimate with each other. Maybe you can surprise her with one of our massage aids to show that you support their new dedication as a couple!

Truly,
Patty

"Let's Talk about Sex, Baby"

I can almost hear you saying: "Okay, date night is one thing, but communicating about sex is another matter entirely." For so many couples, just the idea of talking about sex is embarrassing. For many men and women who have grown up with mixed and distorted messages about sexuality, the notion of having an open dialogue with their sexual partner can make them freeze up with anxiety. Anxiety and fear lead to avoidance, and what happens next? Problems go untended. The void between partners deepens. Desire gets buried. And all the while, golden opportunities for closeness and passion are missed.

Bringing your reenergized connection into your sex life is a very personal, individual process. There isn't a fail-safe formula that works for everyone. (How many of us have said, "Honey, we need to talk," and yet how many of us have cringed at the idea of saying, "Honey, we need to talk . . . about sex"?) Together, though, you and your partner can find the path toward intimate communication that feels right to you.

You may be a couple that already feels comfortable being explicit about sex. Many couples find this kind of sexy talk exciting and use it naturally as part of their foreplay. If this isn't your style, there are plenty of other ways to connect with your lover without needing to get graphic or explicit. For example, I often suggest to couples that they create a code for talking about sex, a private shorthand that lets them reach out to the other and show interest without having to be explicit. As a couple, you might come up with a code phrase that signals you're in the mood. Think of it as an invitation for a little romp at the end of a long day. Something like—"I'd love to have wine and cheese for dinner tonight, how about you?"—could do just fine to let your partner know, simply and without a lot of fuss, that you're interested. After all, as I like to say, "Sex doesn't have to be about fine dining every night; some nights, wine, cheese, and crackers works just fine."

Be Positive

Talking to each other about sex starts with being positive. Remember the "comfort zone" I talked about in Chapter 1? You've been working on creating that nonjudgmental, positive, open space in your own mind where it's okay to be curious about your sexuality, where it's okay to acknowledge the things that turn you on and stimulate your mind and body. Now it's time to extend that comfort zone to include your partner.

Let each other know that you're interested in spicing up your sex life, or that you want some changes. These initial conversations, sometimes just simple acknowledgments of your desire to become more sexually active and in tune with each other, can go a long way toward taking the taboo out of talking about sex with your partner. I've found that when couples recognize their mutual desire to be better lovers, they begin the process of being more open and accepting of sex in general. When one woman, Kim, finally admitted to herself and then told her partner Matt that she was bored, "it was like a giant balloon burst in the room. Both of us were bored—now we're trying things and actively talking about sex. It's fun!"

Tell Him It Feels Good

An important part of communicating with your partner involves being able to tell each other what feels good. Since you've been paying special attention to what arouses and stimulates your body, let him in on what you've learned! When you're feeling close and relaxed, tell him, "I really like it when you kiss me on my neck." If you've discovered that you really like g-spot stimulation, then ask him, "This feels great, can you try it?" Be honest, be direct, and use positive, affirming language. Most of us want to be able to talk about sex in bed, but it just doesn't come to us naturally. So I always advise starting with the basics—"I love it when you touch me there" or "I love it when you do this." You can also indicate your pleasure—or discomfort—using body language.

Ask Him What He Likes

From here, it's a natural next step to ask your partner what he likes. Is there something new that he'd like to try? Remember, the goal here is to be open to whatever is on each other's mind. So listen carefully, and give your partner your full attention. If he suggests something new and unfamiliar, and your initial reaction is negative or judgmental, hold your tongue. Don't rush to dismiss his idea just because it's different. These tips are all about becoming open to trying new things, so if you both are willing to experiment, then go for it. Now is the time when trust and acceptance, those hallmarks of strong communication that you've been working on outside the bedroom, can really serve you. And remember to be patient with both yourself and your partner. Developing a vocabulary for talking about your sexual life takes time, and it's not going to feel perfectly natural or comfortable overnight. But believe me, it will happen more quickly than you can imagine! Then again, if talking turns you on, then go for it. All of us like to hear that we are doing something right—we like the reassurance of knowing we are good lovers. This feedback makes our performance better.

When It Doesn't Feel Right

It is also important to be able to tell your partner when something *doesn't* feel good. If something hurts during sex, you need to be able to tell your partner, without embarrassment or fear of hurting his feelings. If you're feeling any pain or discomfort during lovemaking, speak up. In the trusting, open climate you're creating as a couple, this is important information for you to share, and for him to understand.

Intimacy Issue #5—"I'm embarrassed to talk about sex."

Carol wrote to me saying that at thirty-two she was afraid to talk about what she wants sexually. I asked her if it was a problem with libido and she said no. Instead, she confessed that she felt uncomfortable talking with her husband. I told her that too often we forget the basics of communication, so I suggested that she and her husband play a game: Write out on separate pieces of paper five romantic or sexual things to try for five nights straight; toss the pieces of paper in a hat; and then choose one each night to explore. If Carol and her husband played the game with an open and accepting attitude, I bet they were laughing and loving in no time. You can, too.

Are you young and single? Lucky you! Now is the time to start building your communication skills. Just as a financial planner will tell you to start saving right now for your long-term economic health, I'm here to tell you that it's never too early to learn to communicate honestly and openly about sex, as a foundation for a lifetime of emotional and physical well-being. As always, the first step begins inside you. Whenever you're embarking on a new relationship, amid the tingling excitement and the cascading nerves and the surging emotions (and hormones!), *stop* and ask yourself: What do I want? Am I ready for this relationship to become sexual? Give yourself permission to really reflect on these questions, to take the time to answer them fully and honestly. There are simply no wrong answers to these questions, only answers that are right for you in this particular time and place in your life. There is no formula that tells us when it's time to become intimate with another person. The best thing you can do for yourself is to learn how to listen to your mind and your body, and to use that information to clearly express your own wishes and desires. And when you do become sexually involved—communicate, communicate, communicate! In learning how to ask for what you want, how to share your likes and dislikes, and how to encourage your partner to open up as well, you position yourself for a lifetime of healthy, fulfilling sexual experiences. Imagine the kind of wonderful relationship you can build with your partner if you employ these communication techniques right from the start.

Closing a Gap

For couples facing serious illness, a move, or some other life-changing event, strong communication skills and a healthy relationship can truly serve as a lifeline. Yet when physical or emotional challenges arise, we often shut down—especially with those we are closest to. Any kind of crisis at home or work can put extra strain on a couple's relationship, but with understanding and awareness, such difficult times can also bring a couple closer together. Your sexual relationship can survive and even thrive despite a crisis.

Debra is one of the many incredible, brave women I know who are winning their fight against breast cancer. Diagnosed in 1999 just two months before her forty-fifth birthday, Debra, a young wife and mother, went through a grueling series of treatments to combat her cancer, including radiation, two rounds of chemotherapy, and a partial mastectomy. Debra told me how, amidst the stress and fatigue of her illness, and the side effects of treatment, she and her husband managed to reconnect emotionally and sexually: "I can vividly remember my wonderful husband making a romantic overture one night and I said to him, 'I am fat, bald, and mutilated. How can you possibly want to make love to me?' His reply: 'You are my wife and in my eyes, you will always be beautiful.'" Debra found life, hope, love, and, yes, a full and deeply satisfying sex life in the wake of breast cancer, and so can you. (See Resources section)

Another woman's story hit even closer to home. Nancy (her real name) has been a dear friend of mine for years. When she had reached five years remission with Hodgkin's disease, she invited me and some other friends to go out and celebrate. During the evening Nancy had clinked champagne glasses and truly enjoyed herself. Then later that evening in my car she broke down crying, saying "Do you know when I was going through my treatment, my husband wouldn't touch me? He showed absolutely no interest in me. It made me feel horrible."

Gently, I asked if she had asked him to touch her or be intimate with her, and she said no. She assumed he would have known that's what she wanted.

Following that evening, Nancy went back and asked her husband. And what did he say? He thought that if he pressured her for sex or intimacy, he would hinder her recovery. What a terrible loss came from that lack of communication. Thankfully Nancy and her husband were able to reconnect emotionally and physically.

If you need your partner to hold you, you need to communicate that need or desire. For instance, you could try saying, "I need you to sleep next to me." We often look to our partners to be "mind readers," expecting them to know exactly what we want or need. Instead, you need to show or tell your partner what those needs are.

Strong communication is the absolute cornerstone of a healthy relationship. Learning how to communicate with your partner about your sex life is just one part of the puzzle; you must also take a look at how you and your partner communicate in all ways, not just in the bedroom. Finding ways to connect, to share your thoughts and feelings, making time to spend together in activities you both enjoy, and sharing an ability to express love in thoughtful words and deeds are habits of couples who make communication a top priority and do it well. With these skills, you and your partner will be able to nurture and maintain a relationship that will keep you physically and emotionally connected for a lifetime. Pillow talk is important! Expressing your desires to your partner, and listening as he expresses his, will reenergize your lovemaking in ways you can't imagine—that is, until you ask! So get talking!

CHAPTER SIX

"Your Body Is a Wonderland"

Discovering the Power of Touch

ONE OF THE most powerful ways to build intimacy is through touch. Of all our senses, touch is the one that connects us most immediately and tangibly with another person. A loving, gentle touch between two people can serve so many purposes. Touching one another makes for great foreplay in the bedroom; it also keeps couples emotionally connected, and helps us keep our brains connected to our sexual pulse.

In addition to the emotional benefits of touch between partners, physical contact—particularly in the form of massage—offers some pretty powerful health benefits as well. Many studies show the health benefits of touch and massage in improving sleep, lowering stress and anxiety, and boosting feelings of relaxation and well-being that extend far beyond the time the touching actually occurs. Being touched and massaged can help combat fatigue and give you more energy. Studies also have shown that massage gives a demonstrable boost to the body's immune system. One such study tested the effects of massage on women diagnosed with Stage I or II breast cancer. The results were dramatic, including a reduction in depressed moods, anger, and anxiety among the women. The longer-term benefits were even more astounding. After receiving thirty-minute massages three times a week for five weeks, the women's immune systems were producing more of the natural killer cells to combat disease, as well as making more of the body's own natural painkillers. Another study conducted on patients with chronic fatigue syndrome found similar results: Regular massage resulted in less pain, better sleep, decreased anxiety, fewer stress hormones, and more pain-killing, mood-lifting hormones.

There are a number of physiological forces at work here, as our bodies respond to touch in several important ways. A positive, pleasing touch causes the body to release endorphins, powerful natural chemicals that flood the body with feelings of wellness. When the body is under stress, or battling anxiety, it releases hormones, such as cortisol, that increase blood pressure and actually suppress the immune system. Touch and massage not only bring stress levels down (thereby reducing the amount of cortisol in the body), they also stimulate the immune system itself, triggering your body's own natural defense cells, which work to clear the body of toxins and ward off disease. Just imagine: While you're getting lovingly stroked on the outside of your body, enjoying the sensation of being touched by your partner, inside, your cells are being mobilized and energized to work better at keeping you healthy. This is definitely a win-win scenario: something that feels good, and also is good for you! And yet so many couples have shared with me that the longer they are together, the less affectionate they are.

Falling Out of "Touch"

Think back to when you and your partner were first together. You probably couldn't keep your hands off each other, right? When you weren't tearing each other's clothes off, you were thinking about it. And even when you weren't in the bedroom (or wherever else you found to be intimate), you probably spent a lot of time just touching each other. Maybe you treated each other to massages, maybe you sat on his lap, rubbed each other's back, snuggled close together. You probably didn't have to remind yourself to be close with your partner; it just came naturally. After all, when you're falling in love, reaching out to touch the object of your affection is all you want to do.

Somewhere along the line, for many couples, that impulse gets buried. We've all heard of the "honeymoon phase," those thrilling, tingling, wildly sexy times early in a relationship when lust and romance are everything, when you can't get enough of each other, when the feelings of falling in love, and being in love, override almost everything else in your lives. It is a common and natural progression to eventually move out of this lusty, romantic phase toward a different kind of balance in your relationship, one marked by a deep attachment. But frequently, when the honeymoon phase passes, it carries with it the physical closeness in a relationship, leaving couples adrift from each other, sexually and emotionally. Just as the sexy underwear you used to wear gets shoved to the back of the drawer, the special, sensual kinds of touch that used to be constants in your relationship get pushed aside.

Claire and Bill are a perfect example. Married for nine years, with three children, the couple regularly puts in sixteen-hour days running their family's restaurant business and taking care of their kids. When I first met Claire, she felt miles apart from Bill, both physically and emotionally. The first few years of their marriage had felt charmed, she told me. "We had so much fun together, looking back it feels like we were always laughing about something, just happy to be together."

But the demands of daily life, of parenting and running a business, making time for family and friends, had taken its toll. Claire mourned the deep, close, romantic relationship she once enjoyed with Bill, and she felt at a loss as to how to turn things around. I asked her about their sex life, and I also asked whether or not she and Bill made a habit of touching each other, both inside and outside the bedroom. She thought about it for a long moment. "We used to be so touchy-feely with each other," Claire told me, "but somewhere along the way we just sort of stopped." I suggested she start by reaching out in the simplest ways to make physical contact with her husband, as a way to begin the process of reconnecting. We also went over some suggestions for waking up their communication—for often when couples stop talking, they stop touching.

I also recommended that each of them create a wish list of things they like in the relationship, as well as changes they thought would make them happier and bring them closer. When they shared their lists with each other, and when they put aside time for more regular date nights (for more suggestions see Calendar of Connections in Chapter 9), Bill and Claire began a gradual process of reconnecting.

When I ran into Claire a couple of months later, she rushed up to me, her face flushed with excitement. Things had clearly taken a turn for the better.

"I remember the first time I reached out and grabbed Bill's hand while we were driving to work," she said. "He looked at me so surprised, and then he gave me the biggest grin. Now he takes *my* hand all the time!" For Claire and Bill, getting back into a routine of touching opened a door to reconnecting at a deeper level. "We're not any less busy," she said, "but I feel like we're checking in with each other more, even if it's just by a quick kiss or a squeeze."

You may think you're doing what you have to do, tending to all your responsibilities and obligations. You may think that putting the health of your relationship in the backseat, so to speak, is an unavoidable consequence of your busy life. But there is a demonstrated link between the quality of our sex lives, our physical closeness with our partners, and our basic level of contentment and fulfillment. One recent study looked at happiness in relation to both money and sex. Surprise! They found that more sex makes us happier than more money. Economists who interpreted the data equated a happy, sexually active marriage with the same level of happiness resulting from $100,000 annual bonus! (Think about *that* the next time you or your partner is deciding whether to work late.) Some researchers believe that the secret underlying this happiness-sex connection is—you guessed it—touch. Couples who are regularly engaging in sex are, naturally, touching each other on a regular basis, and it's that regular dose of positive physical contact, with all its physical and psychological benefits, that makes us happier. If you've lost this vital physical closeness with your partner understanding the reasons why is important, and it's also important to begin working to restore that intimacy.

For couples finding their way back to intimacy and reigniting their physical passion, tender moments of physical contact—reaching out to hold your partner's hand or a simple massage to rediscover what feels good about touching and being touched—are essential. These moments are also an important part of the process of renewing your bonds of communication and trust. Exploring each other physically and getting reacquainted with your bodies (and I mean the entire body, not just those obvious erogenous zones!), will bring you closer together. In sharing this sensual, intimate time, you'll literally be putting yourselves in another's hands, allowing yourselves to be vulnerable and open—all experiences that can bring about a forceful resurgence of trust.

ASK PATTY:
Erogenous Zones

Dear Patty,

What are erogenous zones? Where are they on the body? Are they different for men and women? Thank you!

Searching for Pleasure

Dear Searching for Pleasure,

The term "erogenous zone" describes a number of places on the human body that are highly sensitive to touch. Every person has his or her own hot spots and the best part of foreplay is discovering these spots on your partner.

In general the most sensitive body parts include the nipples, lips, scrotum, glans (head) of the penis, the clitoris, and the vaginal lips. However, many people also find touching the earlobes, back of the neck, inside of the thighs, and small of the back highly sensitive. If you want to find all of your partner's erogenous zones, use our Dust Me Pink edible body powder on your partner. Couple it with a blindfold so your partner has to concentrate on the areas that feel good to him or her. You will know when you have hit a new erogenous area! You can also use the Erotic Massage Manual and the Aura Massage Oil to guide you to new places or old favorites with new techniques. Don't forget to let your partner make some discoveries on you too!

Truly,

Patty

Getting Started with Massage

For many couples, taking those first steps toward intimacy can be awkward and nerve-wracking. When you've fallen out of practice touching each other, it can be scary to start over again. Maybe you're afraid you've forgotten how. Maybe you're worried he won't like what you do. Maybe you're nervous about sharing with him what *you* want for the first time. When I advise couples that are struggling to reconnect sexually, I often suggest that they start by massaging each other. This simple yet highly erotic interaction warms the skin and muscles, arouses the body, and awakens erogenous zones you didn't even know—or had forgotten—you have! It's a great way to reintroduce yourselves to each other, and to all the pleasures of being close.

When Massage Is Unfamiliar

I'm constantly surprised when I find people who don't like massage—or at least they think they don't. To many, massage seems unfamiliar. People may not think about incorporating massage into their romantic routine, or they're reluctant to try, simply because they're afraid they won't know how to do it properly. There is nothing difficult about giving a great massage, and a few simple techniques and tools can make massage both easier for the giver and more pleasurable for the receiver. Massage is not about using a complicated technique. The art of massage is all about spending time with your lover, slowing down, and learning how to enjoy the sensual experience of touch.

The Wonder Massage

It is perfectly okay to give a massage with your bare hands, if you prefer, but I recommend that couples try using a massage glove. The Pure Romance Super Deluxe Mitten has long, soft nubs on one side and small, hard nubs on the other side, so you can vary how you apply pressure, intensity, and type of sensation. Imagine that the glove is a natural extension of your hand.

Especially for people who feel nervous or tentative about experimenting with massage, a glove can help facilitate touching, making the "work" of massage a whole lot easier. It's also a way of saying to your partner, "I'd like to make a change in the bedroom." The glove heightens the sensation of a massage, and reduces some of the effort for the massage giver. What more could you ask?

Whether you use a massage glove or just your hands, I heartily recommend using massage oil or lotion (Pure Romance's Ro-

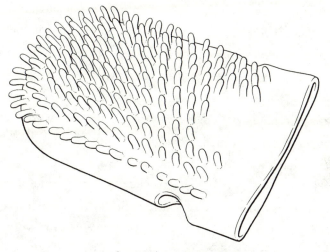

Super Deluxe Mitten

mantica), which can be applied directly on the glove. Massage oils and lotions serve to lubricate and make it easier to rub the skin. They also provide a warming sensation, which is both relaxing and stimulating. Massage oils and lotions come in any number of scents (and tastes!), so you can easily find one that appeals to you and your partner. Experimenting with a selection of oils and lotions in search of your favorites can become part of the fun!

Now, I'm not interested in helping you settle for just an ordinary sex life, so I'm not going to give you instructions for just an ordinary massage. My famous, sure-to-bring-zing-to-the-bedroom massage involves a massage glove and a vibrator. You'll be amazed at how this little toy can transform your massage from *run-of-the-mill* to *oh-my-goodness*! I suggest using a vibrator as part of a massage to increase the wow factor (it's also a great way to introduce a toy into your relationship in a gentle, nonthreatening manner).

In this leisurely, sensual massage, you and your partner will be touching each other from head to toe, awakening all your body's erogenous zones along the way. You'll be concentrating on the non-sexual parts of each other's bodies—because remember, ladies, erogenous zones are not restricted to your privates! Your back, your arms, hands, legs, and feet can all be erogenous zones. Desire and arousal are stimulated in many ways and places, and this massage is all about getting reacquainted with each other's entire body and expanding the realm of what it means to turn each other on.

Here's how it works. The vibrator goes inside the massage glove, and provides wonderful stimulation everywhere it touches your partner's body, without you having to do all the work. Believe me, when you see how much fun this is for both of you, you'll want to have some energy left over when the massaging is done! Start by having your partner lie facedown. Starting at the nape of the neck, begin a gentle massage with slow, circular, sensuous strokes. From there, work slowly down and across your partner's back, shoulders, and arms. As you make your way down his back, you can even massage the top of his buttocks. (Or, to delay pleasure even longer, skip over the buttocks.) Work your way down each leg, from thigh to calf, and spend some time gently massaging the feet. When you have thoroughly covered your partner's back side, ask him to flip over. Beginning again at the neck, gradually massage his shoulders, chest, and arms. Massage his legs, from top to bottom. Rub his ankles and the tops of his feet. The goal here is to cover every bit of your partner's body, while slowly discovering what pleases him and how pleasurable it is to be touching each other.

Resist the impulse to rush! Soak up the wonderful smell of the massage oil, enjoy the softness of your partner's skin, and luxuriate in the warmth you're generating simply with your touch. As you caress your partner, notice what especially stimulates him, whether it's a specific spot on his body or a certain kind of massage stroke. As a couple, you will be developing a repertoire of touch and a variety of practices that you know you'll enjoy together, and learning each other's favorite ways to be stimulated and aroused is an important part of the process.

Now it's your turn to be on the receiving end of a sensual, long-lasting massage. At this point, your partner is relaxed and, we hope, appreciative of your efforts. With a little luck he has learned a few things from your attentiveness to his body. Let him take over the vibrator and glove, and don't be afraid to guide him—help him get started, let him know what feels good, and where else you'd like him to touch you. Remember to keep your feedback positive and encouraging as you communicate your desires.

With this massage, you are adding new dimensions to your intimate, physical relationship. You're learning how to be free, to take your time, to focus on the pleasurable sensations of the moment. You're learning how to be mindful of what makes each other feel good. You've also found a way to bring a toy into your bedroom without a lot of nervous fuss, and together you can decide how you might like to use this toy for other types of fun.

ASK PATTY:
Rendezvous Reluctance

Dear Patty,

My fiancé will soon be returning home from a long trip overseas, having been gone for six months. I want to do something really nice to make the reunion extra special. Do you have any ideas on how to romance him off his feet? He really appreciates these romantic gestures from me and I know he deserves them for all that he's done. I'm not sure I know how to give a massage, but I'm willing to learn. Any suggestions on what the most sensual massage lotion/oil would be? Also, how should I go about setting up our bedroom? We've both been dreaming about this night for a really long time and I just want it to be perfect.

Thank you,
Reluctant with Our Rendezvous

Dear Reluctant with Our Rendezvous,

Wow! What an exciting time for you and your fiancé! You definitely came to the right place. I'm glad to be able to help you set the mood and enhance your intimate nights, whether it is a romantic homecoming or part of your weekly routine. You'll definitely want to invest in some massage oil or lotion. There are so many types and scents available that you'll want to try a few to find out your favorites. (I'm sure your fiancé won't mind testing them out with you!) Then, after you feel really comfortable with your massage skills, I would recommend setting the mood in your bedroom. Dim the lights, and try using a linen spray infused with pheromones to enhance your sexual scent. Don't be afraid to be dramatic— throw a bunch of rose petals on your bed! You can also light candles to introduce a soft glow and sensual mood to your room. There are a few other things you can include to insure that the massage will

*not be the last activity of the night. One is a soy
candle. Light the candle and let some of the candle
melt, blow out the flame then pour it directly onto
your lover. Soy melts at a very low temperature, so
there is no risk of being burned by hot wax. You can
then indulge in the soft, warm body oil by massaging
and rubbing it onto your fiancé's skin. It only takes a
few drops to do a whole body massage! Need a
little twist? Trying giving your massage with a
personal massager, which will add stimulation and
relieve you of some of the work! Enjoy!*

Truly,

Patty

Setting the Scene for Romance

Wouldn't it be great to enjoy the sensual pleasure of your massage in a luxurious environment? While a special weekend getaway can be a wonderful treat for couples, you and your partner don't have to spend a lot of money traveling to a spa resort in order to bring some extra pampering and sensuality into your love life. It's easy and inexpensive to bring "spa treatments" right into your bedroom, and expand how you massage and touch. Bringing the feel of a spa into your home just takes a little planning and creativity.

When arranging your bedroom rendezvous, it's worthwhile to think about creating an atmosphere that stimulates all your senses. Creating a romantic environment also can help put you both at ease while you're getting used to this new type of intimate exploration. Scented candles and aromatic oils can play with your sense of smell, and when you dim your regular lights, candlelight can transform the look of your bedroom into a glowing, romantic setting. (As for sense of taste, well, just you wait; we'll deal with that in a minute!) Here's a great trick: How about lighting a candle that is made of soy? Soy candles burn at a very low temperature, which allows them to serve more than one purpose. As your soy candle burns, the oil will melt into a warm liquid, and you have instant massage oil!

We all have linen closets stocked with sensible, everyday sheets for our beds. Rather than pulling out the same pajamas you sleep in every night, give yourself permission to splurge on something new and indulgent that you and your partner can use on your special nights. How about some new lingerie? In advance of your massage night, pick up a set of sheets in your favorite color in a soft, Egyptian cotton, or even a slippery silk! Also, make sure you keep a ready supply of your favorite bath and shower gels, soaps, and oils on hand. Set aside enough time so you can take a steamy shower or bath before you and your partner get started. This will leave you feeling relaxed, smelling fantastic, and ready to be close and playful with your lover.

So, are you interested in taking this playful, sensuous touching experiment a step further? Here's a fun massage game, with a tasty twist. You'll need to include a couple of simple aids: a feather teaser and an edible body powder. (For information on where to find these products, consult our website www.pureromance.com.) With these toys, you and your partner can indulge in sexy, touching play that will engage all your senses. Use the feather to dust trails of powder all over your partner's body. With your mouth and tongue, go back over the dusted trail and nibble or kiss away! Be sure to pay close attention to what drives him crazy because you'll want to remember it for the next time. Now, let him dust you. If you'd like to spice things up even more, you might want to try incorporating a blindfold into your bedroom activities. Taking away your sense of sight will intensify your other senses, and help you focus more completely on the stimulation of the feather teaser and your partner's touch. A game like this is likely to lead you two into some pretty hot places!

Staying in the Moment

Okay, so clearly massage can be a terrific form of foreplay—but it's important to remember that massage doesn't always have to be a lead-in for sex. A lot of men tend to assume that a massage will automatically result in intercourse. Sometimes it can, and sometimes it does. But I encounter many women who feel that once they start something sensual in the bedroom, like a playful massage, they are then obligated to have sex.

Ladies, rid yourselves of this idea! Nothing could be further from the truth. It's always up to you whether or not you want to progress from touching to something more intense. Hey, you might get really turned on and carried away, and before you know it, your massage has turned into foreplay. If so, great! But you are under no obligation to get hot and heavy if you're not in the mood. I want couples to use massage to slow down and make time to explore each other, to learn how to be in the moment, without jumping ahead to a sexual conclusion. When it comes to building a deeply satisfying sexual life with your partner, it is all about learning how to fully enjoy every moment of the journey—and not race ahead to a particular destination.

If your man is like most of his kind, then you might have to lead the way here, and teach him how to slow down, stay in the moment, and stop fast-forwarding to what may—or may not—come later. My friend Rita went through exactly this with her husband Tom. For several months, Rita had been frustrated by her lack of interest in sex. We talked a lot about the reasons why her libido might be diminished, and one of the things we came up was the pressure she felt about the whole situation. Initially, Rita liked the idea of introducing massage into their bedroom activities, but every time Tom touched her, or she felt like touching him, she would start to worry and feel pressure about whether or not she would want to "go all the way." Tom, on the other hand, would try to make the most of any opportunity for intimacy with his wife by moving too quickly from massaging to sex, which of course only made Rita feel more pressure! These two were stuck in a difficult, lonely cycle.

The breakthrough came when Rita was able to communicate to her husband that she needed to experience this time of sensual play without worrying about where it was leading. That very night, they made a pact: To take sex off the table for a while, and let massage time be just massage time. No matter what, they decided, they would focus on the massage itself, and not let things progress to having sex. This allowed them both to experience their massage nights in a new, lighthearted manner. She stopped feeling pressured. He learned to slow down. Before too long, they were renegotiating that no-sex rule!

"It seemed like kind of a crazy thing, to decide not to have sex when not having sex was our problem," Rita laughed. "But it turned out to be a great step for us. Now we are both able to enjoy things as they happen, whatever that means on any given night."

Troubles with Touching

Why is touch so awkward and difficult for so many of us? In some cases, women who don't have a positive body image feel uncomfortable being touched—even in a nonsexual way. It's no secret that we're fixated on weight and appearance in this country, and that the media directed at women promote a single body type (think tall and thin with large breasts and a small waist) as the one and only ideal. Look around you—we know this is pure marketing, but many of us harbor insecurities about our bodies that cause us to feel bad about ourselves and to not want to be touched, even by our most trusted, intimate partner.

Women tend to pick their bodies apart mercilessly, looking at each piece of their physical selves separately—and critically. "My boobs are too small" or "My hips are too wide." One thing that can help is to try to think of, and live with, your body as a whole, integrated unit, rather than a series of parts you either like or don't like. Stop focusing on your thighs long enough to see yourself—all of yourself—and realize that you're a pretty terrific package!

A serious illness can threaten and profoundly alter a woman's body image, her perception of herself as a physical person, and her willingness to be touched by her partner. Maggie is one of the many women I know who has confronted this issue. Maggie took on her fight with cancer with an incredible spirit and attitude, and a wonderful sense of humor. During her treatment, she found ways to look stylish with colorful, zany scarves, and she bragged about her new "perky boobs" after her reconstruction surgery. If anyone were going to get through the ordeal of breast cancer with her positive attitude intact, it would be Maggie. And yet, she struggled with the image of her post-cancer body.

"You see," she told me, "after breast cancer, you tend to lose more than just your breasts. I'll never forget the day that I took the bandages off for the very first time. That is one scary image! One look and you turn *yourself* off, and you are convinced that you will never turn anyone else on again. You are convinced that your sexual self is gone."

Maggie found help among a community of women where she could talk about her fears and also her desires, and she now shares that support with other women. "When someone gives you permission to be a sexual creature again," she said, "Wow, what a wake-up call."

And sometimes, a woman who can barely stand to be touched may have been abused in the past. A history of physical and/or sexual violence can understandably make a woman fearful or reluctant to be touched, even when she's moved on to a supportive, safe relationship. (In such cases, it's important to seek professional help; reach out to AASECT, a national organization that can recommend a sex therapist in your area.) In other cases, women (and men, too) simply are unaccustomed to being touched by loved ones. For those of us who were raised in homes without much physical affection, getting into the habit of touching and being touched by our partner is a major life change.

Intimacy Issue #6—"I don't like to be touched" or "I don't like my body."

In talking to thousands of women about their sexual hang-ups every day of the year for the last twenty-five years, it's still surprising to discover that many women don't like to be touched. Some might have experienced roughness or abuse in their past. Some may never have been touched—even as children. Some fear touch because they have such low self-esteem and poor body image that the mere thought of being touched makes them recoil.

For example, the women I've worked with who are recovering from breast cancer are often afraid of touch because they have become insecure about their body image. Together, we work on reestablishing a sense of positive body image through touch. The touch itself becomes a means of healing.

For most people, a bit of knowledge and instruction, together with positive exploration, tends to alleviate nervousness and anxiety about being touched. Sharing your body with another person is always your decision and you have to grow into that comfort zone. If you are afraid of being touched in a nonsexual way or you avoid this kind of interaction with your partner, you may want to seek professional help. (Contact AASECT, WWW.AASECT.ORG.)

The power of touch to enhance and transform your relationship—and your health—is immense. Making a physical connection with your partner is an important step toward revitalizing your sexual and emotional life together. You want sizzle in the bedroom? Make time for a massage (with fun, tasty tools), and watch as the sparks begin to fly again. Sensual touching and massage can actually add new dimensions to your intimate relationship; it's a form of foreplay, a way to expand your knowledge of each other's erogenous zones, and a way to grow more connected as a couple.

If you're tempted to try massage but nervous about moving too fast, too soon, remember that *you* determine the pace in your bedroom. Let your lover know what speed feels right to you, and together the two of you can take your time getting to know each other's bodies again. You don't need to worry about what might or might not happen afterward; being fully present for a sensual, loving massage is its own reward. Any kind of touch creates the need and desire for more intimacy, and like a chain reaction, will lead to only more pleasure.

CHAPTER SEVEN

Pure Pleasure

Lubrication Education

EVERYONE SHOULD HAVE a good lubricant. Period. Yes, you can have sex without one, but why should you? Would you brush your teeth without toothpaste? Would you skip your conditioner if your hair was dry and brittle? If you truly want to be a good lover and maximize your experience in the bedroom, then lubricants, in all their many forms, are the answer.

Although lubricants have been on the market for many years, many women are not yet aware of how great these products are at enhancing intercourse and other types of sexual play. Made for internal and external lubrication of the vagina, penis, and anus, lubricants are the easiest way to make all sorts of sexual play, including intercourse and masturbation, more comfortable for both a woman and her partner. Lubricants also help relieve the dryness that so many women experience during sexual activity, even when they are aroused. Many women find that a lubricant actually helps with libido problems, by reducing pain and discomfort and stimulating their desire or triggering their arousal. Specialty lubricants enhance pleasure and stimulation, assuring that all your sexual play is pain free, safe, and nothing but pleasurable fun.

Many people make assumptions about lubricants that are based on misconceptions or the wrong fit. Introducing a lubricant during sexual play is quite simply a wonderful, enhancing bonus, once you've found one that really works for you. Like finding a comfortable, supportive bra or a shampoo that adds volume instead of flattening your fine hair, you have to spend some time to educate yourself about the options and then decide what's best for you (and your partner).

And yet, despite these tremendous benefits, I can't even begin to tell you how many women I've met who've never even considered using a lubricant. And I've met countless others who are stubbornly resistant to the idea. What's up? Let's start with a little lubrication education.

Clarifying Misconceptions

A common misconception is this: If you're not experiencing self-lubrication naturally, then you are not excited or aroused—or worse yet, there is something wrong with you. Ladies, believe me when I tell you, this simply is not true! So before we look at the array of options, let's take a look again at what happens to our bodies when they get aroused.

It is true that a woman's body naturally becomes lubricated when she's aroused. However, there are a host of factors that can affect your body's ability to naturally lubricate, ranging from temporary to chronic, mild to severe. As mentioned in earlier chapters, any number of medications you take may inhibit your body's lubrication, including allergy and cold medicines and also many antidepressants. Lifestyle choices, such as diet and exercise (particularly extremely rigorous exercise) can dehydrate your body, including those membranes that would naturally lubricate when aroused. So can cigarette smoking, giving you yet another reason to quit if you currently smoke. Having a baby can affect your body's ability to create its own lubrication; the same is true for when you're nursing. Women coping with serious or chronic illnesses—cancer, immune disorders—often experience difficulty with lubrication. And menopause (because of reduced estrogen levels) is in itself a leading cause of vaginal dryness, pain, and discomfort—all of which result from a decrease in the body's ability to self-lubricate.

During sex play, other factors can also influence a woman's natural lubrication. Feeling stressed out or pressured will affect your body this way, as will a lack of arousal. During intercourse, being penetrated before you're ready can impede self-lubrication. Do you recall Colleen's harrowing story? In retrospect, it was clear to her that had she known to use a lubricant, her injury might have been prevented. With or without these factors in play, many women's bodies simply do not always produce enough moisture to last the duration of intimacy. It comes down to this: no matter how excited you are, it's good to use a lubricant.

And yet, for all these factors lessening our natural lubrication, many women assume that using a lubricant means there's something lacking with their own bodies or the state of their sex lives. As Marty put it, "I've always felt that if I used a lubricant, it meant that something was wrong with me." And Lori said, "Using a lubricant meant that I am a bad lover."

So despite all evidence to the contrary, some women with

whom I've spoken have actually shared that they feel inferior or inadequate if they think they have to use a lubricant. For those of you who also feel this way, let me tell you this: Our vaginas are not meant to be in a constant state of openness, ready for penetration. Therefore, it is important to give your body the time or the tools it needs to prepare for penetration. Think of it this way: You use a moisturizer on your skin, right? You probably pay special attention to certain parts of your body, such as your face and your hands. And you've likely noticed that there have been times during your life—certain times of the year, certain times of the month, during pregnancy, or menopause—when you've experienced extra dryness in these places. I'm willing to bet that you have never put yourself down for using a moisturizer, or believed there was something wrong with you or your body because your skin is sometimes dry! Well, the more sensitive areas of your body are no different, and the right lubricant can serve the same gentle, hydrating purpose as that jar of face cream that's sitting on your bathroom sink.

Like a lot of women I meet, Jennifer harbored these sorts of reservations about using a lubricant. As new parents of a lively infant daughter, Jennifer and her husband were in the process of adjusting to life post-baby. The good news was that both of them were excited about resuming their sex life, and eager to spend loving, intimate time together. The not-so-good news was that Jennifer was discovering a few of those little secrets of motherhood that nobody ever seems to share—about how pregnancy and childbirth can affect a woman's body, and even change the notion of what normal means, in terms of sex. "I mean, forget how everything looks different with your body," she confided to me one night after a Pure Romance party. "Things also really *feel* different."

One of the differences for Jennifer was a decrease in her body's ability to self-lubricate. She'd listened to the fun, free-wheeling talk among the women at the toy party. She'd heard all the talk about the wonders of lubricants, how they can make sex more pleasurable for both women and men. But when I gently inquired about whether she and her husband were using one, she stiffened.

"I just feel like that's giving in to the problem," she lamented. "I mean, I never had to use one before."

I gently probed, "Giving in? Can you tell me what you mean by that? Do you think this is a contest?" I explained that there was no "problem" with her body at all, nor with her desire for her husband. She simply was experiencing a natural change in the way things work with her body. By the time we finished talking, I had managed to extract a promise from Jennifer to at least consider trying a lubricant. A couple of weeks went by and I received a lovely email—from none other than Jennifer.

> "Dear Patty," she wrote. "Wow, do I feel silly for making such a fuss. In this case, I am VERY HAPPY to admit I was wrong!"

Intimacy Issue # 7—"Ever since I hit fifty, I am all dried up."

Sex during and after menopause need not be any less fulfilling than it was before—in fact, with a little knowledge and support on your side, it can be even better! There's no question, menopause can bring big changes—and many times, challenges—for our bodies and our sex lives. Did you know that 80 percent of postmenopausal women experience some type of sexual dysfunction? Vaginal dryness, fluctuating hormones, decreased blood flow to the pelvic area, and even night sweats can decrease sexual desire! Also, during menopause, the walls of the vagina can become thin and tender, making sex painful. Finding a lubricant that works for you can be an important part of your health regimen both during and after menopause.

For women who have reached menopause, we recommend that a woman use a vaginal moisturizer 2–3 times per week. We also recommend that she use a water-based lubricant during intimate moments (when she is with a partner, using a bedroom accessory, or is simply pleasuring herself). Although a water-based lubricant may dry out more quickly than a silicone lubricant, a water-based lubricant will actually absorb into the skin and help counteract some of the negative side effects of dryness, much like keeping hydrated and using lotion can benefit your skin. We also recommend the importance of Kegel exercising. By promoting a healthy vagina through moisture and exercise, women can oftentimes overcome the dryness permanently.

However, when extreme dryness is a chronic problem and a vaginal moisturizer and water-based lubricant help, but aren't enough, we also recommend adding a silicone-based lubricant into the routine. For information on managing your sexual health during and after menopause see the Resources section.

A Little Gift

Unlike Jennifer, Faye was immediately open to the idea of using a lubricant. Her concern was with her husband, Jerry. After twenty years together, Faye and Jerry had weathered some of life's challenges—the deaths of their parents, financial worries, several moves as a result of Jerry's job—by turning to each other for support, and they felt very bonded as a couple.

Faye loved Jerry, and he loved her—they still said it to each other every day. "It's part of our morning and evening routine," Faye said, smiling proudly. But things in their bedroom had grown *too* routine. Moreover, Faye had reached menopause about a year ago, and she was experiencing a mild decrease in libido, as well as some persistent dryness. Using a lubricant seemed to be the perfect remedy, and Faye was all for it.

But she was nervous about introducing something new into their bedroom. In particular, she was afraid her husband would take her use of a lubricant as a slight against him. "I just know him, and he is definitely capable of feeling really insecure about sex. I'm afraid he'll take it the wrong way, and think it means there's something wrong with him."

I let her in on a little secret: She was not alone in this concern. It is incredibly common for women to feel some nervousness about introducing anything new to their intimate routines, especially if they feel their partners may resist. I reassured Faye that she was capable of introducing this new element to their bedroom in a positive, affirming way, without hurting her husband's feelings. "After all," I reminded her, "You're doing this because you want your sex life to be even better, which is a great compliment to him."

We talked about how to raise the subject, how she could share with her husband what she had learned about her health and her body, and also share with him her desire to make a positive change in their sex life. We brainstormed some good analogies for her to present to him (toothpaste, hair conditioner, etc.) in a light and humorous way if she needed to. Faye thought the one that worked best would be something that her husband could relate to: "Using a lubricant is like adding oil to your car to make the engine run better."

Armed with her new knowledge (and the lubricant that was right for her, one that was tasteless and odorless), Faye was ready to make this change for herself. After their next sexual encounter, wouldn't you know, Faye's husband surprised her! Far from being hurt or offended, he was relieved to know that she'd found a product that could help her feel better. He was supportive of her desire to take control of her sexual health and well-being, and, as Faye herself said to me with a giggle, "he was a little turned on by the whole thing!"

Later on, I ran into Faye at another party and she told me how much more pleasurable and enjoyable their sex life was for both of them. Without the pressure created by the dryness, she was so much more relaxed. She told me that now their favorite place to make love is in the shower! Of course, I suggested she use a silicone-based lubricant so it will last in the shower, and she can continue to enjoy herself.

Most important, Faye herself has been thrilled with how the lubricant has worked for her. "Taking care of the dryness problem has made me feel so much better, and I think it's helped with my desire level, in general. Knowing that sex is not going to be uncomfortable makes a big difference."

As with any aspect of your intimate life, open communication is key. You need to work at being honest with your partner about how you are feeling, what your body needs, and why you want to make a change to your bedroom routine. (Hint: Because you love each other and want to be sexy and close!) In my experience, I've found that fear of a partner's reluctance turns out to be overblown in the end, as most partners are happy to do a little experimenting. Guys like spice and variety as much as we do!

However, some women are truly uncomfortable bringing up the subject. If you are a bit reluctant to discuss the matter with your partner, I suggest simply using a dab of tasteless, odorless, water-based lubricant before you plan on being intimate; they tend to work for hours, and your partner will never need to know!

I will let you in on a little secret: some men think that when a woman is not wet something is wrong, that she doesn't love him anymore or that she may be thinking of someone else. Men can make assumptions that something is wrong in the relationship even if the reason you're dry and not responding in your typical manner is just stress. That's when you might consider going into the bathroom and applying a little dab of lubricant. And when you're intimate, you might just hear, "Oh honey, did I do that for you?" Let it be a little gift from you to him.

ASK PATTY:
Dry as a Desert

Dear Patty,

Lately I have been in the mood to be intimate, but once my partner and I begin foreplay I become extremely dry. Is there anything I can do to help my lubrication problem? Thank you.

Dry as a Desert

Dear Dry as a Desert,

First, it is important to figure out if maybe medications you are taking are adding to your lack of lubrication. Are you taking any type of antihistamine, birth control pills, diet pills, or an antidepressant? If so, you may want to check with your health care provider, as any of these medications could be causing the problem. Stress, menopause, and your diet could also be contributing to your vaginal dryness.

We suggest starting with a mild water-based lubricant that is most like a woman's own natural lubrications. This product should be used during intercourse or with the use of a bedroom toy to maximize your arousal while adding the lubrication necessary for effective stimulation. If you find that the lubricant is working, but it doesn't feel like enough, you may want to integrate a vaginal moisturizer into your routine.

Just remember, you should always make sure that if you are engaging in intimate activities, you should enjoy them!

Truly,
Patty

Welcome to "Lubrication 101"

Ladies, there is life beyond KY! When I travel around the country, educating women about all topics sexual, one of my favorite ice-breakers is showing women the many wonders of lubricants. As I've said, there are many types of lubricants to choose from and I know without a doubt that you can find the one you are meant to enjoy. Lubricants don't just help remedy dryness and discomfort, they really do enhance the sensations of intercourse and other types of sexual play. And since there are oh-so-many ways to play around with your lover, there are also many types of lubricants! Sometimes I find that women can be confused, and a little overwhelmed, by the variety of lubricants available out there. The easiest way to explain this is to think about the assortment of common personal products you use everyday—things like that moisturizer I spoke about earlier. If you're like me, you have your absolute favorite brand of shampoo and you change your brand from winter to summer. (And you always make sure to buy more before you run out!) You also probably use the same deodorant time after time, because you know it works for you. You've chosen to invest in makeup that suits your complexion as well as your lifestyle. Sometimes we change and sometimes our bodies need something new. Also, sometimes people don't like lubricants because they use too much and it becomes messy. Remember, all you need to use is a nickel-size dollop on yourself and on him.

Your own body chemistry also affects the types of lubricant that are best for you. We all have our own unique sensitivities and preferences. Some of us have oily skin; some of us have dry skin. Some are prone to allergies or are extra sensitive to scents. And others enjoy scents—especially fruit, vanilla, or lavender. Moreover, these sensitivities and preferences inevitably change over time and as our lifestyles change. You're probably using a whole different set of personal products now than you were ten or twenty years ago. Well, lubricants are no different than any other common personal product! You'll probably want to change them too, after a while.

Lubricants can be found in an array of colors, textures, and flavors. In my work, researching, educating, and developing intimate products for women and their partners, I recommend two main types of lubricants for regular, sustained use: water-based and silicone-based. To supplement these everyday lubricants, I've also spent time developing what I like to call "playful lubricants," which include warming lubricants, which bring a little extra heat to the bedroom, and creamy lubricants, which are especially good for you to use on your man! These are not designed to replace your everyday, water-based lubricant, but they can bring a sexy dose of spice and variety to your intimate routines. It's the difference between your everyday stylish slides and a sexy pair of stilettos!

ASK PATTY:
Do Vaseline and Bedroom Accessories Work Together?

Hi Patty,

I do not have lubricant and I only remember that I need it when that moment arrives. Is it safe to use Vaseline with my Pure Romance toy? Thank you, Forgetful

Dear Forgetful,

Vaseline shouldn't be harmful to your Pure Romance toy, but it is definitely not good for your vagina (or for condoms). The oil in the Vaseline can break down latex condoms, causing tears and possible breakage. Do not use Vaseline as a lubricant when using latex condoms during sexual activity. Because Vaseline is oil-based, it is not as healthy for your vagina as a water-based, or silicone-based lubricant. Vaseline may cause infections and irritation because the oil in the product causes it to "linger" in the vagina longer than a water-based or silicone-based lubricant. To be on the safe side, I recommend using a water-based lubricant (silicone-based lubricants should not be used with silicone toys, as the lubrication will break down the toy). Just Like Me is a great water-based lubricant that isn't sticky and is very gentle.

If your toy is not made of silicone and you prefer a silicone-based lubricant, I recommend Pure Pleasure. Silicone-based lubricants are best to use for water activities and during anal play. Both Just Like Me and Pure Pleasure are safe to use with latex condoms. I would buy a bottle of lubricant to keep on hand for whenever the moment arrives!

Have fun!

Truly,
Patty

Everyday Lubricants

It's important to have a lubricant that you can use on a regular basis, whether it's for intercourse, sexual play, or self-pleasure. This lubricant should be gentle and sensitive to your body as it works with your own natural lubrication. (You should never experience irritation, pain, or discomfort with your lubricant.) It should also enhance your sexual pleasure, and help eliminate any discomfort that comes with dryness. As you now know, there are many times in a woman's life when outside factors can impact how well her body is able to produce its own natural lubrication.

Whether for short or long periods of time, whether because of medication, stress, or life-altering events like childbirth or menopause, there simply will be times in every woman's life when her body may not be able to produce a sufficient amount of lubrication.

For everyday, I recommend choosing a product that is water-based and water-soluble. Water-based lubricants are easily absorbed by the body. After all, the human body is made up of roughly 55 to 65 percent water! A water-based lubricant is a safe, reliable, and gentle choice for most women. When you are aroused, a water-based lubricant will work with your body to give you a mild rewetting quality. These lubricants will often dry out during extended sex, but they can be easily reactivated with a small amount of your body's own lubrication, with water, or with saliva.

Water-based lubricants are a good choice as a starting point for women who are just beginning to experiment with lubricants. "I felt weird about using a lubricant at first," said Jodi, a twenty-two-year-old student. "I wasn't wild about the idea of using something that wasn't natural to my body. But the lubricant I found is really gentle, it makes everything go very smoothly! And I don't really even notice it, after I've applied it."

You can use water-based, water-soluble lubricants on a daily basis, and they are safe for your body to use over the long term. They are also safe to use with both latex and polyurethane condoms, as well as all other types of barrier birth control, such as diaphragms, contraceptive sponges, cervical caps, and the "female condom." These lubricants are very gentle in combination with your body, and are extremely unlikely to cause any irritation. And here's a bonus—not only will a water-based lubricant not irritate, but regular use of water-based lubricants can actually reduce the *symptoms* of vaginal dryness, which include itching, burning, and irritation.

Lubricants made with water will be compatible with most bedroom toys, which is another big plus when you're looking to add some variety to your sex life! (For more information on which lubricants to use with specific toys, see Chapter 8.) Water-based and water-soluble lubricants score high points for versatility and effectiveness, and as a result they are the type of lubricant that health care providers tend to recommend most frequently as a safe, reliable choice for women.

But wait, just because water-based lubricants are trusty and reliable doesn't mean they have to be boring! There is plenty of variety to keep you and your partner busy trying these lubricants until you find one (or a few) that you like. You'll find these lubricants in liquid and gel form, so play around to find out which texture you prefer. Also, if you want to be just a little bit adventurous, lubricants actually come in flavors! At my company, Pure Romance, we make a couple of flavored water-based lubricants— we have one that's strawberry flavored—and I'm telling you, I hear lots of great feedback about these "tasty" products. If you're naturally sensitive, though, you might want to stick with an unflavored lubricant. And just so you know, even unflavored lubricants will taste a little bit sweet, because of the composition of ingredients. You and your lover can have a lot of fun finding out just what your tastes are, when it comes to an everyday lubricant.

> ## Warning
>
> Always read the ingredients to make sure a product doesn't contain oil—some water-based products can still contain oil and therefore cannot be used with a condom; oils break down latex, and decrease the condom's protectiveness.

Silicone-Based Lubricants

If you and your partner like to get sexy under the sea—or in the tub or the pool—then a silicone-based lubricant is just what you're looking for! Silicone-based lubricants can be used similarly to water-based lubricants, but they have one big difference: silicone-based lubricants are completely waterproof, making them ideal for underwater use. They also last longer than water-based lubricants. Because the silicone molecules in the lubricant are too large to be absorbed by the skin, they become highly concentrated on the skin's surface. So in this case, a little lubricant goes a long way! The ideal amount for you to use is no larger than a nickel; this amount will enhance your pleasure for a long time, whether you are in or out of the water.

Their high concentration also makes silicone-based lubricants the safest lubricants to use for any anal love-making. Because the rectum does not lubricate naturally like the vagina, any anal stimulation requires a long-lasting lubricant for added safety. If you and your partner enjoy anal play, then it's important to use a silicone lubricant. These lubricants are safe to use with latex condoms, and we strongly encourage using a condom for any type of anal penetration, to avoid spreading bacteria.

We're going to talk about toys in Chapter 8, but it is important for you to know that silicone-based lubricants are not compatible with bedroom toys made from silicone. Remember from your high-school chemistry class that "like dissolves like"? Silicone lubricants will break down silicone toys, creating larger pores to harbor bacteria in the toy. You should use a water-based lubricant if you are using silicone toys. An alternative is to cover your silicone toys with a latex condom before using your silicone-based lubricant. Like water-based lubricants, silicone-based lubricants are compatible with both latex and polyurethane condoms. When you're choosing a lubricant, you always want to make sure that it's compatible with any other bedroom accessories you plan to use. It's a great idea to have several on hand, so you and your lover can be as spontaneous as you want with your sexual play!

Using a vaginal moisturizer such as Fresh Start, in addition to a water-based lubricant, can be helpful for women who are in any of the stages of menopause, as well as in women who are coping with age-related dryness that occurs more often than just during intercourse. This was exactly the case for Andrea, a vibrant woman in her sixties. When I met her, she was struggling with both a low libido and an irritating dryness that made sex painful, and also persisted apart from intercourse. We talked about her particular needs and circumstances and decided that she begin by using a product such as Fresh Start (a vaginal moisturizer) to rehydrate her, and then introduce a water-based lubricant to counteract the dryness. You don't want to mask a problem, and it's a natural part of aging to lose moisture. Again, you wouldn't think about going to bed without putting on moisturizer on your face—your vagina wants and needs this same kind of replenishment. If the dryness does not seem to lessen, try adding a small amount of silicone lubricant in addition to the vaginal moisturizer and water-based lubricant. The same is true right after you've had a baby; your vagina is extra dry and needs to recover its natural balance of moisture. Andrea found relief from the dryness and pain, and feels she's making progress with her libido. "I still struggle with desire, and sometimes it's hard for me to get started with sex," she said. "I'm not always 'in the mood' as much as I'd like to be. But using a lubricant has helped me. Sex feels better, and I'm not feeling the pain that I used to. I'm getting used to the idea that sex can just feel good again."

Playful Lubricants

Okay, so you've got a closet full of everyday clothes, a rotation of reliable ensembles that you can throw on in a hurry when you're rushing to get ready in the morning. Then, somewhere tucked in the back of your closet, is *the dress*. Maybe it's glittery and shiny and really short, maybe it's long and elegant and velvety; whatever the style, when you wear it, you feel like a movie star. You'd never want to put it on everyday—imagine vacuuming your living room or doing household chores in that very same dress—but on special occasions, it sure works to make you feel great, and your partner probably gets a thrill from it, too.

Well, try thinking of the lubricants you use in a similar way. No, really! You're going to have at least one gentle, mild lubricant—but hopefully a selection—that you can use as often as you'd like. And then, you'll want something a little more . . . special. This is where "playful lubricants" come into play. These lubricants can be made of water-based or silicone-based materials—at Pure Romance, we make ours water-based—but whatever their basic composition, they contain additional properties and ingredients that can change both the consistency and the function of the lubricant. These changes are designed to take pleasure and stimulation to a whole new level. (Remember, it is not safe to use them with condoms, because the flavorings have oil that breaks down latex condoms and toys.)

Mary Beth, thirty-two, was feeling reluctant when her boyfriend asked her to give him oral sex. Like many women, she was afraid to "taste and smell him so closely." As women, we like to be in control of what we put in our mouths, and what can help women in this situation is to use something familiar, such as an edible lubricant that tastes pleasant or fruity. In Mary Beth's case, I suggested she use Lickity Stiff, which has the added benefit of being a heightener too!

Playful lubricants are perfect for giving an extra thrill to activities such as oral favors, self-stimulation, and erotic massages. They make foreplay so much fun, you'll be rushing to turn off the television and dive under the covers. In my work over the past two decades, I've focused my attention on two of the most effective of these types of lubricants: *warming lubricants* and *creamy lubricants*. Each has its own special properties and best uses.

Warming Lubricants

Warming lubricants are great during foreplay, as they are designed to heighten arousal and sensation. When a warming lubricant is rubbed on the skin, it does just what its name suggests: it creates heat, flooding the area with warmth, delivering pleasing, stimulating results for you or your partner. If you apply additional friction to the lubricant—or use your warm breath—the lubricant will continue to heat up, providing even more stimulation! When you're just beginning to experiment with a warming lubricant, you'll want to start small. Gently rub a dime-sized amount into a small area of the skin, applying more as necessary. As you continue to massage, the lubricant will begin to heat up, causing your partner to feel a pleasantly warm sensation. Because of the intensity of the stimulation, warming lubricants are meant to be used in modest amounts and not intended for full-body massages. Warming lubricants are great for genital massage, oral favors, or for massaging concentrated areas of the body, such as the breasts or buttocks.

Some warming lubricants contain oils and cannot be used with latex products, so make sure to read the label before using (again, oil breaks down latex). Like water-based and silicone-based lubricants, warming lubricants come in a range of delicious flavors, as well as unflavored versions. For those of you who enjoy receiving oral favors, but maybe don't love giving them, this is a product that can take away some of the work, while making everything taste amazing.

For women who have used regular lubricants, branching out and trying these playful aids can be an exciting way to broaden your bedroom *repertoire*. "I had never experimented with a lubricant beyond what they distributed at my doctor's office," said Tracy. "I started using it in my twenties. I just always needed a little help if sex went on for a while. But I never even thought about whether there were other kinds of lubricants." After attending a Pure Romance party with some friends, Tracy decided to try a few other types of lubricants, including a warming lubricant. "It's pretty amazing, the stimulation you get, and I mean both of you," she said. "My boyfriend gets really turned on when he sees how much *I* like it. And vice versa! We have a few different kinds that we like, so we rotate using them, to keep things fresh."

If you're like Tracy, and have already been using a lubricant, then maybe it's time to try something new. If you're new to the world of lubricant, there's no reason to wait. These warming lubricants are beginner-friendly!

Creamy Lubricants

The other type of playful lubricant that I find effective and attractive to the women I meet is what are known as creamy lubricants. Creamy lubricants not only enhance love-making, they can help make the experience extremely comfortable for both partners. These lubricants have a thick, emollient texture, which can provide long-lasting lubrication. They are also wonderful lubricants to use with a number of bedroom accessories, particularly those that are designed to work on your guy! (Be patient, we'll be talking all about those fun toys very soon!) Men tend to use products like hand or body lotion when masturbating—they like it because it provides lasting lubrication. Whipped is a great alternative for him, or when you want to pleasure your man or when it comes to any toy that encompasses the penis. The creamy lubricant is also good for oral pleasure, for women especially; it's more playful because it tastes good and lasts longer. You wouldn't have a strawberry sundae every day, but on certain occasions it can be a special treat.

Quick Lubricant Tips

Both warming lubricants and creamy lubricants contain oils and cannot be used with latex products. Polyurethane condoms are made of plastic, and do not react to oil-based lubricants in the same way that latex condoms do. Check the ingredients of your lubricant before choosing a condom. Always read your labels and plan accordingly, to make sure you are using products that are compatible. There are also flavored creamy lubricants available. However, women who are prone to vaginal irritation or infections should avoid any kind of product with flavorings—Our Pink Ribbon line, for instance, is made for more sensitive women. In fact, our Pink Ribbon line was created under the recommendation of several gynecologists, nurses, therapists, and even cancer survivors to help with an unmet need for products that are safe for sensitive women without the added color, odor, or flavoring. These women may find themselves easily irritated by fragrances in products like laundry detergents or perfumes. They may also find that they are extremely susceptible to yeast or bacterial infections due to the types of underwear they wear, from taking bubble baths, or even after being sexually active. Some women, like those going through cancer treatments, find that the added colors, odors, and flavors can be irritating, due to their suppressed immune systems.

You're now fully initiated into the wonders of lubricants! Congratulations on incorporating a simple, safe addition into your intimate routine, one that can have tremendous results. (Please visit www.pureromance.com for further information about lubricants.) Whatever life stage you're in, whatever your relationship status, finding the best types of lubricants for you is a major step in your journey to make the most of your experiences as a sexual person. Remember, your needs will inevitably change, so keep an open mind and keep experimenting—what works for you today may change down the road. It's not so important what kind of lubricants you choose, but that you pay attention to your body, be aware of your likes and dislikes, and share these with your partner. Together, the two of you can find the selection of products that suit your needs, and are compatible with your other toys and aids. And don't hesitate to investigate on your own!

CHAPTER EIGHT

Batteries Not Included

The World of Toys

EDROOM TOYS ARE an exciting way to add new sensation, spontaneity, and new paths of sensual pleasure. When
you and your partner introduce this playful element to your relationship your sexual energy will increase with gusto! As Mike and
Sharon said to me, "We never knew that toys were going to be so
much fun. They make us feel young and giddy again. They are so
freeing!"

"We never knew . . ." I can't count the number of times I've
heard this from people who have come to enjoy the pleasure and
excitement of bedroom toys. Many people simply have never
given toys a second thought. Others are afraid of the idea of bringing a toy into their bedroom. For two decades, I've been helping
people break through their fear of the unknown to enter the sexy,
playful world of "grown-up" fun.

Finding Your Comfort Zone, Again

I can guess what some of you might be thinking: Sounds good, but toys are for other people—more adventurous people, richer city people, younger people—anybody but me and my partner! In my work, what I do more than any other single thing is talk to women. Over the years, I've spoken with thousands of women: regular women, who drive carpool and attend PTA meetings, who belong to garden clubs and organize church events. Believe me, if you're thinking you'd like to experiment a little with a bedroom accessory to make your sex life more interesting and change it up a bit, then you are not alone! Thousands of women out there feel just as you do. Over and over again, I've had the pleasure of seeing people find freedom and a new sense of themselves once they follow their desires. Something wonderful happens to people when they let go, move out of their old comfort zones and tired routines, and allow themselves to play and explore with their sexuality, and bedroom toys can be a great way to do this. But often, this comes after they've overcome deep-seated reluctance and fear.

Most women come into a Pure Romance party thinking they'd never use a bedroom toy. They project an attitude of "There's not one thing for me here," and can almost seem defensive. But I promise you, it's usually those women who end up in my Ordering Room saying, "I can't believe you made me feel so comfortable with this!" or "My partner's fantasy is to watch me pleasure myself, and this toy will make it so much easier" or "Your demonstration shed a whole new light on what these products are all about."

The reason for reluctance that comes up most frequently is

that "nice women" don't use toys. Wives and mothers, this thinking goes, shouldn't engage in such behaviors. Well, what behavior
are we talking about, exactly? Embracing the fullness of your
identity as a sexual person, for the sake of your health and happiness? Following through on your desire to have a lively, sexual relationship with your partner, and be sexually fulfilled as an
individual? Admitting that despite all the responsibilities in your
life, you still just like to have fun, and you deserve to be able to
devote some time and energy to grown-up play? I think you'll see
that this notion that "nice women don't play with bedroom toys"
is rooted in those old judgments about sex that so many women
and men were raised with: messages that sex is bad or wrong, and
that enjoying sex—really taking pleasure from it—makes you
somehow less of a "good girl."

"It was really hard for me to let go of the idea of toys being
kind of wrong," said Jamie. "I really had to look at all my attitudes
about sex, and how I thought about it from the time I was a kid.
Once I started to do that, it was like everything started to change.
When I realized I could choose to think differently about sexuality, it gave me such a powerful feeling. After that kind of change,
I thought, 'Toys, why not?!' "

A lot of women have found themselves through *Sex and the
City*—watching that show, women learned it was okay to try a
bedroom toy because Carrie Bradshaw and her friends said so. At
Pure Romance parties, I've often overheard, "Oh, you have one?
So do I!" The affirmation, relief, and a sense of belonging are all
present in their voices. And you don't have to worry—your interest in or desire to try one will not be branded on you like some
kind of scarlet letter—this is a private choice, and one that you
alone can share with your partner or use on your own.

Another all-too-common resistance to toys stems from a fear, on the part of one partner, that bringing accessories to the bedroom is a message that he or she is doing something wrong, or is lacking in intimate skills. This happens more than you can imagine. One way to overcome this reluctance is to communicate your interest in toys as a part of your interest in your partner. The message becomes "You are sexy and make me want to play," instead of "I need something to play with since you're not very sexy." A lot of times when women say to me "I've never owned a bedroom toy, but I want to buy one—what should I get?" I tell them to book a party where they can touch, taste, and test the products firsthand. If a party isn't convenient, then go online. The idea is to educate yourself and become familiar with your options. If I were simply to list our products, you might not ever try a bedroom accessory. But when you can spend time looking at the specific toys (see below) and really think about what might appeal to you and/or your partner—then you are much more likely to try one.

Others worry that once they bring a toy into their bedroom, it will work a little too well! I've met plenty of men and women who feared that their new toys would outperform them. There is no toy that can replace the human touch, much less the bond created between lovers. Toys are about introducing new sensations and novelty. They help both women and men explore the full range of their sexual desires and ability to experience pleasure. Toys are always—and only—meant to enhance your lovemaking and sexual play, never to crowd out or overshadow a lover. I like to say that men are like microwaves and women are like crockpots: women need time to warm up, while men can come to a boil almost instantly! For this reason, using toys during intercourse can help take the heat and pressure off of him, while helping you to get nice and warmed up! And if you are now single, toys are a wonderful way to stay in touch with your sensuality—take advantage of the pleasure a toy can bring and don't give up on intimacy just because you don't have a partner!

As you can see, a lot of these fears about toys stem from a general lack of confidence in the bedroom. This is why positive communication is so crucial, especially when you've decided to suggest trying something new. The way you choose to bring up the subject of toys, or how he brings this up with you, will greatly affect how you respond to the proposed change, and how much you're able to enjoy the experimenting. The irony is, successful experiences with toys actually make people feel more confident with each other, and with their intimate skills. There's nothing like seeing your partner get excited to boost your confidence!

Sometimes, I find, despite all reassurance, people are just afraid of trying something different. Afraid of not being "normal." Afraid of how something new will feel—and worried they won't like it. The most important thing to remember is that you are in control: it's up to you to decide when and how you'll use any toy. If something doesn't feel right, stop. If you're not enjoying yourself, say so. Make an adjustment. Try a new position, or a different activity. The unknown can be frightening, but there are great rewards for those who are willing to venture in search of new experiences. Not everything here will necessarily appeal to you: the point is to be open to the things that do sound fun, exciting, and appealing. Trust yourself enough to do this.

Remember, too, that your body might not respond right away to using a toy. Often women have to try them several times before they understand how to use them and how their bodies respond to them. This is why, as I've said above, it's a good idea to try one on your own first—so you know how to use it and what types of toys really work best for you. Some can take a toy home and achieve that wow factor right away. Others need more time—you have to find what suits you best.

Introducing Toys to Your Partner

I truly believe that the most powerful words in the bedroom are "I would like it if . . ." Simple statements of desire that begin like this are a nonconfrontational, nondemanding way to open a dialogue with your partner about making all sorts of changes in the bedroom, and toys are no exception. When your partner understands that your desire to bring something new to the bedroom is about finding new ways to appreciate each other—and *not* about being deficient in some way—he or she is much more likely to react positively. But you need to be clear and direct. Don't assume that your partner knows and understands your motives. You will be paving the way for a smooth introduction of toys or any new element to your intimate life if you go out of your way to let him or her know that "I love you and I think you're sexy, and I'd love for us to try this together." You can bring the subject up casually, maybe during a long drive. Perhaps say something like, "Have you ever thought about trying a bedroom toy?" The idea is to raise the subject in a nonthreatening way—as something that might *add* pleasure to your relationship.

I know a lot of women like Madeleine, who struggled with how to communicate her interest in toys to a reluctant husband. Madeleine wasn't afraid to talk about sex, or shy about the idea of toys. To the contrary, she was so outgoing about her new interest that she overwhelmed her unsuspecting husband! Madeleine was so excited after her Pure Romance party, she rushed home and showed her husband Jim her new vibrator. He reacted negatively.

"I'm not one of those women who can have easy orgasms during sex, and I really thought this would help. I was really hurt when Jim dismissed the idea so quickly."

Madeleine backed off for the time being, but she didn't give up. She took her time, and waited until she had some quiet, private time with her husband when they were both relaxed. "We'd gone away for the weekend to a wedding, and we were in this very romantic spot. We'd had a great day together, just wandering around outside, having lunch, doing stuff we never get to do."

Madeleine brought up the subject again, a little more gently and keeping in mind the affirming, positive attitude that we talked about, and this time Jim agreed to try a massage. "I realized I needed to slow down and explain to him why I wanted to try," Madeleine said.

Over the years of working with so many couples, I have noticed that the partners who seem to maintain the strongest relationships over a long period of time tend to have a broader definition of what intimacy means. One night they may prefer to have intercourse, another night, they will give each other oral favors. Sometimes they add toys, sometimes they engage in mutual self-stimulation, sometimes they play games or just give one another a sensual massage, depending on their mood. The idea is that they like to change things up. They know that varying what they are doing in the bedroom keeps the relationship fresh and exciting.

Since toys can add variety and spice, they can also help bring about positive changes in your relationship and create an enthusiasm that is contagious! It is important to talk to your partner about why you want to add new elements to your sexual relationship. Make sure you reiterate that you find your partner sexy, that you want to touch him in a new way, in order to keep opening up new dimensions to your intimate life together. If you're comfortable, take the time to share with him what you've learned about your body, your libido, and the life cycles of an intimate relationship over the long term. Invite your partner to view your new bedroom toys as you do: a way to open a new chapter in the cycle of your intimate relationship, one that can broaden and deepen not only your pleasure, but also your definition of intimacy itself.

And keep in mind that you don't have to try everything all at once! It's okay to start slowly. In fact, I recommend you do just that. Taking your time will help ensure that you don't do too much, too soon. If one or both of you feels overwhelmed, you might be tempted to give up before you've given yourselves a chance to really explore what toys work for you.

Remember the super deluxe massage mitten with the vibrator from Chapter 6? This is a great first step for couples, a way to bring a couple of new toys into the bedroom without a lot of pressure. After you've grown comfortable with using the vibrator for massage, you can take turns slowly trying out these toys on each other's more sensitive parts. From there, you're on your way.

As you also learned in Chapter 6, finding ways to connect and communicate with your partner about your intimate life will strengthen your trust, whether toys are front and center for a night of play or tucked away in their resting place. All along the way, it's important for you and your partner to keep talking, particularly to keep expressing your affection and desire for each other. Remember, this is a process, and a journey, and the point is to enjoy every step, and make the most of it before embarking on the next one.

Intimacy Issue #8—"I'm afraid that I will become dependent on my vibrator."

Few, if any, studies exist on this phenomenon, but it can be assumed that people do not become addicted to their sex toys. True, people can become addicted to anything, but being comfortable using a toy is not the same thing as being addicted to it. It might be easy for someone to fall into a pattern where they are unable to orgasm without their toy, but by simply changing the way you do things, it won't feel like the same routine. As an easy example, think about the way you work out. A personal trainer would work with you to find an exercise routine that will ensure that your body continues to respond to the exercise. If you maintain the same exercise routine for a long period of time without changing distance, speed, repetition, etc., your body will begin to plateau. It is important to keep challenging your body in order to avoid the monotony you may experience. Arousal can be very similar. If you are trying to become aroused using the same method for a long period of time (the same sexual position, the same speed on a sex toy, etc.) you may notice your body doesn't respond the same way it used to. It may become more difficult to become aroused. It is important, just like with your exercise routine, that you continue to challenge your body and your level of arousal by trying new positions and new ways to stimulate your sensitive areas. This will ensure that you are maximizing your level of potential. Spontaneity is great for your body, whether you are working out in or out of the bedroom.

Before Playing

All your toys should be cleaned when you first purchase them, and before and after every time you use them. If you look at a toy under a microscope, you'll see millions of tiny pores where bacteria can be trapped, so it's very important to clean your toys regularly with a cleaner such as Pure Romance's Come Clean. Using a small amount of our product, wash your accessory in warm water and let air dry or dry with a clean cloth. Keeping your toys clean and sanitized will keep you and your partner safe and healthy, and it also will extend the life of your toys.

Toys for You

As you might imagine, there are several types of vibrators, each designed to serve a specific purpose and bring you a particular sort of pleasure! With all vibrators, as with any toy, you'll want to use the appropriate lubricant. With most vibrators, I recommend using a water-

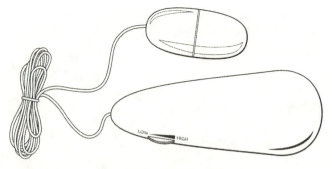

Silver Bullet

or silicone-based lubricant, what you have around for everyday use—remember, products tend to dry you unless you use a lubricant.

Clitoral vibrators are specifically designed to tease a woman's hottest spots! This type of vibrator is a great first toy for women to begin a sexual exploration of themselves, whether on their own or with their partners. The most common type of clitoral vibrator is a small, bullet-shaped toy. These vibrators provide direct vibrations to the clitoris at varying speeds and intensities. Clitoral vibrators allow a level of control, ensuring you get precisely the clitoral pulse you require for attainment of an orgasm. Bullet vibrators tend to be the most common and popular choice among women looking for some help in reaching clitoral orgasms.

Bullet vibrators are also great for massages! You can use your bullet vibrator for releasing tension in the neck, shoulders, lower back, and even the temples (it's so good for sinus relief!). Looking to give your guy an extra-stimulating treat? You can place your bullet vibrator on the outside of your cheek during oral sex for additional sensation to the penis.

As you'll recall, the majority of women experience orgasm from direct clitoral stimulation. Only about one in ten women can orgasm from penetration alone. In addition to using their vibrators for self-pleasure, it is very common for women to use their bullet vibrators during intercourse. Clitoral vibrators are frequently used with c-rings, a male toy that both enhances pleasure and delays ejaculation (see page 197). This way, you both get some playful extra attention!

Some women also enjoy or prefer a nonvibrating toy to stimulate their clitoris or insert vaginally.

G-spot vibrators are designed to target that erotically sensitive area. Both the shape of the toy—an upward-curve—and its vibra-

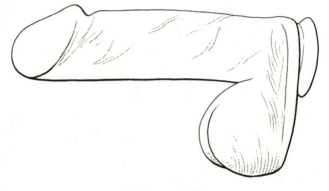

"Mr. Dependable"

tions provide stimulation to a woman's g-spot, which is located on the front wall of the vagina midway between the pubic bone and the cervix. (This area varies in size from a small bean to a half dollar.) Direct stimulation of the g-spot tends to result in quicker and more intense orgasms.

You have to apply some pressure to press through the front muscular wall of your vagina to feel the full effects of g-spot stimulation, which is one reason why g-spot vibrators really come in handy for women who like this kind of stimulation. From the inside, aim your pressure toward your natural pubic hairline on the outside. It sometimes can take a few tries to locate and stimulate your g-spot. Part of the whole process of experimentation is learning to be patient with your body. You'll have a much more positive, enjoyable experience if when you're playing with this kind of toy, you let yourself relax and take your time.

The g-spot becomes more sensitive after you are really aroused, the kind of arousal that comes from clitoral stimulation and orgasm or by lots of foreplay. You may want to continue to stimulate the clitoris as you begin to stimulate the front wall of your vagina.

You can also select a g-spot vibrator that has a multipurpose function. These vibrators have a bullet to simulate the clitoris as well as a curved design for g-spot arousal.

I like to say that multifunction, dual action vibrators are for the woman who has to have it all! These vibrators do a bit of everything, and there are so many options to choose from you can truly customize your sensual experience. These dual action vibrators offer women a variety of sensual experiences during sexual play with a range of options. Typical options for multifunction vibrators include direct clitoral stimulation at varying speeds, a smooth rotating shaft, or a rotating shaft with a variety of beads or ball-bearings. There are also settings for depth and degree of rotation which will affect both g-spot and vaginal stimulation. These dual action vibrators are designed to complement a woman's unique sexual experience.

If you're intimidated by the range of options, keep in mind that you can start slowly, with a simple vibrator. There are beginner-friendly vibrators, usually designed with a slender, tapered shaft, which makes insertion easy, such as the Lean Machine or Hum-

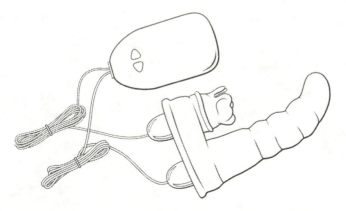

G-Whiz

dinger. With these vibrators, you can experiment with penetration, depending on how you position the toy. And of course, you can use this alone or invite your partner to help you experiment. If you like this type of vibrator, you can eventually move up to a more advanced model, one with lots of bells and whistles! Either way, the beginner friendly options will ready you to move up to such options as the Cowboy Up and Daddy from the 'Nati.

All of these products can help you to achieve orgasm. Your orgasms may feel more intense, may happen more frequently, and may happen more quickly, as a result of using any of these vibrators, alone or in combination with other bedroom toys. But let's not forget: the orgasm isn't everything! Focusing too much on having an orgasm as a measurement of "good sex" can dampen all the fun, and take you out of the moment. As you will see in the next chapter, you want to pay attention to all the wonderful feelings that come with being aroused, and you'll enjoy your sexual play from beginning to end.

Some women are afraid that using a vibrator will cause nerve damage, or desensitize them to stimulation over the long term. Please know that extensive research has found no evidence that vibrators cause any physical harm or desensitization. If a woman holds a vibrator directly on the clitoris for an extended period of

Lean Machine

time, she may temporarily lose sensation (like when your leg falls asleep) but the sensation will return.

What you may notice over time is that using your vibrator may become monotonous. This is true with vibrators just as it is for any other pleasurable act: doing the same thing over and over again can lessen its effectiveness. You probably wouldn't be satisfied with sex in the missionary position only for years and years, and in the same way you may find you need some variety in your vibrators. Try a different type of vibrator—maybe it's time to move from a bullet to something more versatile. You can also use a heightener (arousal cream) with your vibrator, to increase arousal during your play time. Above all else, remember that you're in control of how and when you use your toy. Make the most of the ways it can make you feel good, whether alone or with your partner.

ASK PATTY:
Timid Around Toys

Dear Patty,
  I recently got married, but I have a problem. . . . I am afraid to try new things, like a vibrator. Do you have any suggestions for me?
Thank you!
Timid Around Toys

Dear Timid Around Toys,
  You have done the most difficult thing regarding your fear of trying something new—you asked for help! Great job!

My first recommendation is to start slowly. Don't try to pull out the big guns on the first try. You may find that you aren't ready for it and quit trying altogether! I would suggest use of a small vibrator, to enhance pleasurable sensations through vibration, that can be used alone or with your partner. The *Ultimate 7th Heaven* or *Lean Machine* may suit you best. *Lean Machine* is slightly larger than an ink pen and is not intimidating for first time users. It can be held between the thumb and forefinger so it is easy to incorporate into any massage. To provide stimulation to all areas of the body, simply trace the *Lean Machine* from the nape of the neck slowly down the body pinpointing erogenous zones. This is a great way for a couple to introduce a bedroom toy into a relationship in a comfortable fashion. When you are at ease with *Lean Machine*, slowly try massaging new areas of your body! You will find the fun of vibrators in no time and will be ready for an upgrade.

When you are ready, there are many different options to help you spice things up. This includes everything from lingerie, to books, arousal creams, lubricants, and toys. You may need to do a bit of research on all of your options before you make a decision. And to be honest, www.pureromance.com is the perfect place to discover new things for your relationship, but more importantly for yourself.

Just remember, you have to be comfortable with new experiences, progressing at a rate that feels right to you. Best of luck!

Truly,
Patty

Choosing the Vibrator That's Right For You

Choosing a vibrator is not unlike buying a new car. Think about it. When you're preparing to purchase a car, you consider your options—in the case of a car, things like mileage, comfort, features, and color, what type of driving you'll be doing, what sort of conditions in which you'll be driving.

In the same way, when you choose a vibrator, you want think about what's important to you. The following questions will help you look at your options and decide what type of vibrator makes the most sense for you right now. Take some time to answer these questions, and you'll take the mystery—and the stress—out of purchasing your first vibrator.

What do you want to stimulate? That's the first question I want you to ask yourself. You now know about the basic types of vibrators available, and what types of stimulation they offer. As you're getting to know your body, and paying attention to what stimulates and arouses you, you'll be able to look at your options with a better idea of what type of vibrator makes sense for you, today. Keep in mind, your desires will change and evolve, so you'll likely be choosing to use different vibrators over time.

Think about what type of stimulation you'd most like to concentrate on now—clitoral, vaginal, g-spot, a bit of everything—and work from there. Whether or not you want a vibrator for penetration is a basic initial question. You may discover that in fact you don't enjoy vibration at all and prefer simply the feel of fullness that a nonvibrating bedroom toy offers. This was true of Lysette and George, who we spoke of on p. 120. George enjoyed giving

Lysette oral pleasure while gently teasing her with a toy. There are many ways to include both vibrating and nonvibrating toys in your lovemaking.

How much control do you want over the intensity of stimulation? Every woman's body is different, and will respond uniquely to direct stimulation. Choosing a vibrator with adjustable levels of intensity to suit your preferences is a good idea. Some vibrators (such as PR's Body Rocket) come with removable massage heads, for extra control and versatility.

What type of texture and shape do you want? Well, you've heard it said before: size matters. In this case, I'm talking about the size and shape of your vibrator! Oftentimes, women who are new to the world of toys will feel more comfortable with a smaller vibrator. Whether it's a small bullet for clitoral stimulation or a slender, tapered dual-action vibrator, there are some shapes and sizes that are particularly well suited for beginners.

Do you have a favorite color in mind? Keep in mind, there's nothing frivolous about this. It's a toy, remember? It's a fun, exciting, playful accessory for you to enjoy, whether alone or with your partner. Have some fun with this choice, and select a color that makes you happy or turns you on.

How much do you want to spend? Like so many of our purchases in life, you can spend a little or a lot. Knowing what your budget can handle will help you shop more easily and effectively, amid all the choices available to you. Keep in mind, your needs and interests will change over time, and once you start experimenting with toys, you'll probably want to keep adding to your collection. Starting out with a simple, less expensive toy might make sense, and when you're more familiar with what you really like, you can always invest in something more expensive.

Will you be using your toy in the bath? For so many busy women, bath time is sometimes the only time to grab any real privacy. It's natural for women to want to use this "you" time to fully relax. If this sounds like you, then waterproof toys are the way to go. We've developed waterproof bullet vibrators, as well as dual-action vibrators, g-spot vibrators, and vibrating shower sponges, all perfect for a stimulating soak in the tub.

Many women are concerned about privacy and discretion when they bring their vibrators home. You can ensure your privacy by choosing an inconspicuous-looking toy—smaller vibrators are easier to store and keep out of sight. Also, some vibrators make more noise than others.

Are you going to be travelling with this? Some toys are more subtle than others, such as Pretty in Pink and 7th Heaven. And both of these have an on-and-off button that some women refer to this as the "Oh sh_" button—so if your kids run into the room when you've forgotten to lock your door, you can quickly and quietly stifle the noise of your toy.

Remember, just like buying a car, the more options you want, the more costly the product. And if certain features are important to you (like those of you who can't live without heated seats!), then you're going to pay for them. So if, for instance, you're worried about noise, include "quiet" on your list of preferences. (If you find yourself wanting to purchase a vibrator that is a little noisier, using your toy under the covers or with soft music playing will help muffle the noise.)

Also, take a moment to think about where you'll store your new toy. If privacy is a concern for you, is there a place in your room where you keep personal items, such as a journal or special cards and letters? There are pillows that are made just to secretly stow away your vibrator (like PR's Hide-a-Vibe pillow). These small pillows can be placed on your bed or on a chair in your bedroom. Hard-to-find zippers make this the perfect hiding place for your most intimate treasures.

ASK PATTY:
Ready for Toys?

Dear Patty,

My husband and I are both twenty-eight years old and have been married for five years. We have a great sex life, but I want to spice things up and try new things in the bedroom, like toys and games. The problem is that my husband does not want to try anything new and says we don't need toys or games. What should I do?

Ready to Play Games

Dear Ready to Play Games,

Communication with your partner is key! Some men are apprehensive about using toys in the bedroom because they think they'll be replaced.

I recommend communicating with your partner. Reassure him that he will not be replaced and that this is something fun that the two of you can do together to "spice things up." Because your husband seems apprehensive, I would start out slowly with games. A great way to open the lines of communication is with the help of our dice games, Pair-a-Dice Glow and

Spicy Dice. You can add an additional element of excitement to foreplay by utilizing Dust Me Pink, an edible body powder, that can be traced over any area of the body, turning you and your partner into edible palettes while locating "hot spots" that trigger the location of unknown erogenous zones. An easy way to introduce a nonintimidating toy with vibration into the bedroom is by using the Pulsa Bath Ball during a bath or shower with your partner. You and your partner can give each other a massage by gently guiding the Pulsa Bath Ball all over each other's body to increase arousal and add an effortless massage. This may help your partner become more comfortable with the idea of using a vibrating toy in the bedroom. In addition, remember to communicate with your partner and to take things slowly. Before you know it, he might be bringing in his own toys!

Truly,
Patty

Toys for Him

I'll bet some of you thought that bedroom toys were just for us women! Not at all. There are great products out there that can enhance and prolong arousal and stimulation for men, too. And just like your vibrator, these are toys that you two can use together, doubling your fun. The two most popular toys for guys are c-rings (better known as cock rings), and masturbation sleeves. Both of these toys are best paired with a creamy lubricant, which help make the experience more comfortable and last longer.

The most popular toy for couples to use is the c-ring. C-rings restrict the flow of blood away from the erect penis, creating a pleasurable feeling of tightness and pressure for your guy. C-rings will generally provide men with a bigger, longer erection. They can also help to delay ejaculation, allowing your love making to last that much longer.

C-rings are placed around the base of the man's penis—you may find that it is easiest to put on a c-ring when penis is erect and lubricated, but the best thing is to experiment to find out what works best for you and your partner. The c-ring will fit tightly in a good way; this feeling of tightness and pressure is often very arousing. Some versions of this toy have a double set of rings, one that will fit snugly over the erect penis and the other that will sur-

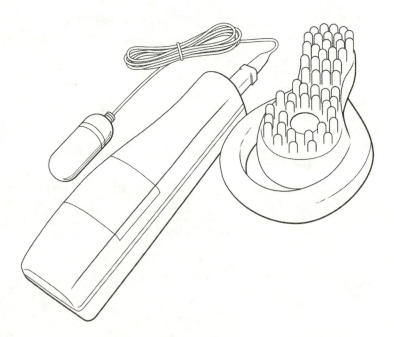

Jelly Tool Belt

round the testicles to hold them in place during intercourse, which can delay his ejaculation.

There are a few things to keep in mind when you and your partner are using a c-ring. This toy should not be worn for more than thirty minutes, and should be removed as soon as it becomes uncomfortable. Your partner may want to trim or shave the hair in the area where he'll be wearing the ring to increase his comfort. And remember to use a creamy lubricant.

Many c-rings have the option to attach a vibrating bullet to them, in order to stimulate the clitoris and/or the anal area during intercourse. (As one person I know said, this "turns the man into a living vibrator!") This is a great arrangement for couples who want to prolong lovemaking for men while also heightening arousal for women, allowing both of you to achieve orgasm. As mentioned, women generally need lots of clitoral stimulation to reach orgasm, and this can sometimes be difficult during intercourse. Very few women can orgasm from a few minutes of thrust-

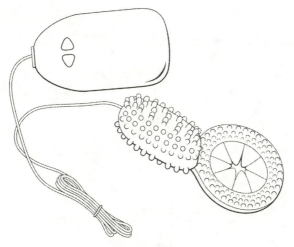

New Jelly C-Ring

ing. Using a c-ring and a vibrator simultaneously can solve this problem of timing and arousal.

Another popular toy for guys is the male masturbation sleeve. Ladies, this is a toy you could buy for your partner for his own use— but keep in mind you can also use it with him! The sleeve provides a degree of control during self-stimulation that many men find exciting and satisfying. Many of them have suction pockets or some other added feature to increase his pleasure, such as beads. The ribbed inside of the sleeve, as well as the pliability of the material, can often seem as real to a man as his partner's own gentle touch. It can also add variety because you can hop on top. And by encompassing the penis, it creates suction, which when incorporated into lovemaking can offer dual stimulation. It's also so slender it can slide into his briefcase and travel with him on long business trips!

Super Stretch is perfect for a partner who is too large or has overwhelming girth. Its open-ended design is great when beginning to experiment with anal play. It can also protect you from total penetration, especially if your man's penis is very large in width or length.

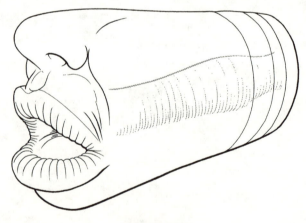

Super Stretch

Anal Toys

Anal toys can be a great tool in helping couples experiment with anal play in a gradual, relaxed, safe—and sexy—way. Keep in mind that the anus is not elastic like the vagina, and penetration may be uncomfortable at first. A small toy, such as a butt plug, can help you get used to the feeling, and allow your body to adjust, before progressing to penile penetration. There are also benzocaine-based desensitizing products (Pure Romance's Booty Eaze), which may help you relax and relieve any pain or discomfort without decreasing pleasure and stimulation. Once you've prepared your body and experimented with gentle penetration, there are more substantial toys you might like to try.

There are several types of probes, both vibrating and nonvibrating, which can provide intense stimulation and also provide a lot of control over the intensity of penetration. Since there is no elasticity to the anus, it's important to use steady motions rather than vigorous thrusting, to help prevent tearing.

Anal beads are another option for couples looking for variety in their anal play. These thin-stranded beads, which are designed

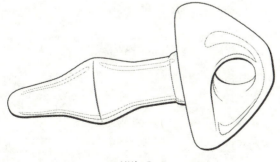

Little Gem

to stimulate the prostate gland from within the rectum, are gently inserted and then slowly removed as a man is achieving orgasm, intensifying his pleasure. (For more discussion on Anal Play, see Chapter 9.)

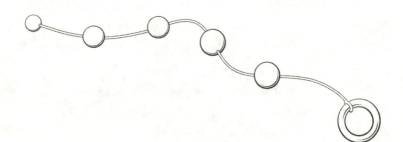

Pleasure Beads

Keeping Things Clean

Playtime is lots of fun, but we always have to clean up at the end! As mentioned above, it's necessary to clean all your toys after every use. To do that properly, you should invest in a cleaner designed specifically for this purpose. Everyday soap and water won't cut it in this case. Regular household soap can damage your toys over time, and the residue is potentially harmful to the delicate tissues of the genitals.

A cleanser specially designed to clean bedroom toys will be gentle to the toy and to the body, and will have antibacterial properties. An all-purpose toy cleaner will be safe on most or all toy materials, such as plastic, silicone, glass, and other synthetic materials. You can rinse your toys with warm water, spray them with cleaner, and rinse again. (Be sure to remove any batteries before you clean your toys!) After you've rinsed your toy, either pat it dry with a clean towel or let it air dry. I recommend storing toys in airtight plastic bags or storage containers. This will keep them clean and in tip-top shape for whenever the spirit moves you to use them! (Visit www.pureromance.com for further information about bedroom accessories.)

Bringing toys into your bedroom can be a life—and libido—changing event for you and your partner. Keeping variety and sex appeal alive makes a profound difference to couples who are trying to keep a relationship vital over the long term. Bedroom toys provide the thrill of the unknown, and can help you continue to see your partner (and he you) in a fresh, sexy, romantic light. Because toys have so much potential for positive changes in your bedroom, it's that much more important to take the time to introduce the idea to your partner with affection, respect, and patience. Toys should never take the place of talking with your partner or working to stay on the same wavelength about your sexual intimacy. But they can bring you closer, as you both explore new boundaries of your sexual desires and capacity for pleasure.

CHAPTER NINE

Moving Beyond Missionary

Expanding Your Pleasure

BY THIS POINT, you probably have come to the conclusion that my approach to sex is all about the journey and not the destination, which is why I've waited until the last chapter to really talk about intercourse. Of course, intercourse can be wonderful, intimate, and very satisfying to couples. But in my experience talking to women around the country, in all age groups and from many different backgrounds, it's clear to me that when too much emphasis is put on intercourse, people tend to rush past all the other ways they can experience pleasure.

And that's the point of this chapter: to suggest a new, bigger way of thinking about intercourse and your sex life in general. I want you to go beyond missionary to find not only positions you haven't tried before but a fresh attitude—one that keeps the importance of intercourse in perspective but enables you to expand your notion of pleasure. The more you can relax and enjoy the ride, the more pleasure you will actually experience during sex. Think of sex as sitting down to enjoy a delicious banquet. You have to open all your five senses in order to truly appreciate all the flavors, scents, and textures, as well as the visual beauty of the food. You need to slow down, stop, and enjoy each bite of the feast. If you rush through the meal, intent only on cleaning your plate, you'll more than likely miss at least one opportunity to discover a new taste, a new slice of deliciousness, and a new sensual experience—and, when it comes to sex, a new way of letting your body enjoy pleasure.

I do offer a brief overview of positions, sharing with you why some couples prefer "going beyond missionary." I also offer my "calendar of connections," a month-by-month guide to enhancing your relationship in ways that increase your intimacy and make you feel more connected to your partner. In a way, this is the ultimate goal of moving beyond missionary: to feel more deeply satisfied and in sync with your lover. If you are now single, by choice or circumstance, you will also find a list of inspirational tips for enjoying being on your own and ideas for joining the dating scene, if that is what you wish.

Opening the Door to Pleasure

Going beyond missionary is all about changing it up, moving out of your comfort zone, and welcoming something new and different into how you approach having sex. Like orgasms, when you shift your point of view from being "intercourse-centric," then you open yourself to discovering that there is a lot to sexual pleasure that does not include intercourse. Sex starts in the head, so that's where we are going to begin.

It Starts in the Head

Since sex starts in the head, it's important to stimulate your imagination. I often suggest that couples pick up a sex book (you will find a great list of titles in the Resource section), go through it together—on a Saturday afternoon, perhaps—and try some of the things it describes. I remember giving a presentation at Ohio State, and encountering a graduate student in his twenties who told me he just happened to come across a book of his girlfriend's that contained creative ideas on how to learn about yourself in a sexual way. Although the book was geared primarily to women, he read it cover to cover and really appreciated all that the book had to say.

A woman, Janet, told me that her husband, a carpenter, was ironically not so good with his hands when it came to touching and pleasuring her. They were in a rut until she shared with him some ideas for new positions that she got from a book. He got really into it—and his hands came to life! Books can really stimulate your brain (see Resource section at the back of the book).

Have Fun!

We all get stuck in patterns, which become boring and dull. We need to jump-start the excitement by making sex fun again. Remember when you were first together and sex was so spontaneous and carefree? It's natural for that "let's-tear-off-our-clothes" feeling to wane once you've been together for a while, but that doesn't mean you can't still be playful in your attitude. You need to make a focused and concerted effort to find inventive ways to add anticipation and energy to your sex life. (Just take a look at all the ways to add this spark in your relationship in the Calendar of Connections!)

Change Your Position

One reason many couples get bored with their sex life is quite simply because they don't change their position. They stick with missionary (man on top) because it's comfortable, fast, and easy, and "does the trick." But when you change your position, even slightly, it forces your body (and your partner's) to make adjustments and you literally create new pathways of feeling. Now, I'm not suggesting that all of you go out and try a position outside your comfort zone. As always, choosing a position for intercourse is very personal—it's totally up to you. But you may want to take a look at these other options and see why some couples prefer or enjoy them.

MALE SUPERIOR—MAN ON TOP (AKA MISSIONARY)

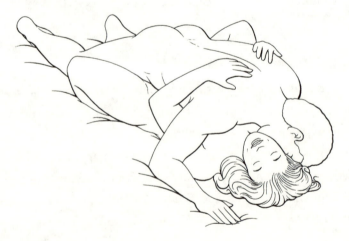

There is a reason many people think of male superior as their standard position: it's easy for the woman, comfortable for the man, and allows for more intimacy because both partners can look at each other. If the woman raises her legs, the man can penetrate her more deeply and some women can better access their g-spot this way. When the man is on top, he can also easily reach the woman's clitoris for manual stimulation—often an added bonus.

FEMALE SUPERIOR (WOMAN ON TOP)

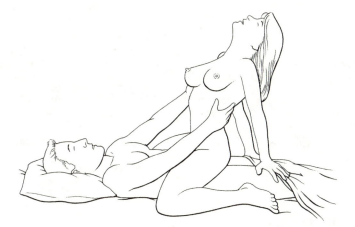

Many women enjoy female superior because they can better control their PC muscles, enabling them to be more in tune with their partner's sexual excitement. As one woman said, "Once I get him excited, I can keep him there for a while." A woman also can control the degree of penetration since she is doing most of the thrusting motion—this is especially helpful for a woman whose partner has a large penis. An alternate way of female superior is when the woman faces away. Some women are able to access their g-spot this way; and some men like this view of her backside.

SIDE BY SIDE

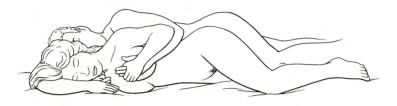

Couples often describe this position as "more relaxing" or "more snuggly." The almost casual intimacy of this position makes couples feel close, and it's also ideal for women who are pregnant or recovering from a hysterectomy. Often the friction is less intense, so climaxing for both partners may take longer—but when you are in the mood for a long afternoon encounter, this may be the perfect position for you.

REAR ENTRY (AKA DOGGIE STYLE)

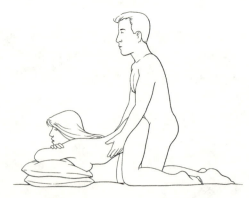

Many men have a strong preference for entering their partner from behind. This more athletic position enables some men to feel a sense of power and physical strength. A man can also enjoy cupping his partner's breasts or stimulate her clitoris quite easily from this vantage point. Many women also enjoy the intensity of penetration they experience with the man behind them. The woman is often able to lead her partner to stimulate her g-spot, and if she is lying down, she can stimulate herself while he is penetrating her.

STANDING/SITTING/KNEELING

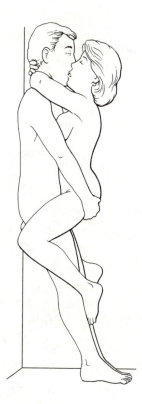

These positions tend to be spontaneous or transitional poses that couples find when they haven't quite planned on having sex, but an encounter seems to develop. A standing or sitting position often uses a prop such as a wall, a chair, a bench, or sofa, which may be why some people who enjoy an occasional sexual encounter in a public place take advantage of these positions. Kneeling is a fun position that often transitions into another position. Check out the Sex Swing and Sex Sling—two great products that add a note of fun.

As you consider all these ways to create new sensation and a new route to pleasure, keep in mind that when you take the risk of introducing something new—a toy, an erotic reading experience, a new position—you not only add spark back into a dull sex life, you revitalize your connection with your partner.

Intimacy Issue #9—"How do I introduce a new position without feeling silly?"

Introducing anything new to a relationship can feel awkward—whether it's about wanting a massage, sharing your curiosity about trying a new bedroom toy, or a desire to introduce a new position into your lovemaking. I always think a gentle suggestion is the best approach. You may want to show your partner *The Complete Manual of Sexual Positions* (see Resources section for full information), and go through the book with him in bed one night. These great visuals of all the different positions will probably get his attention. But if you are sensing he is reluctant or shy because of his body or his ability to hold a position, reassure him by choosing a position, such as female superior, that enables you to do more and him less. The idea, as always, is to be direct about your desires but compassionate about his.

Anal Play

As you first read in Chapter 8, anal play is becoming increasingly popular as more and more people expand their sexual repertoires. Both men and women often enjoy the intense stimulation afforded by the sensitive nerve endings found in the anus, whether by internal or external stimulation, or both. Men may also enjoy the stimulation of the prostate gland during anal play. There are four factors that are critical for safe and enjoyable anal play: protection, communication, relaxation, and lots and lots of lubrication.

I like to say that anal play is a lot like going to a black tie affair. It's not something you do every day, but you spend a lot of time preparing for it. You should be preparing your body and mind each time before you engage in any anal play. Many couples find this a sexy, stimulating way to play in the bedroom, but you should not be pressured into anal sex if you're uncomfortable with it.

Part of what makes anal play difficult or stressful for some people simply has to do with the body's construction. The anal canal has two sphincters, or round muscles, at the entrance. One of the sphincters you can control by squeezing and relaxing the muscles. The other one you cannot control; it will open up only when you are really relaxed. So in preparation for a night of anal pleasure, be sure to take time to relax. Take a warm bubble bath. Spend some time giving each other massages. Enjoy lots of foreplay. When you're ready for anal play and intercourse I suggest using a silicone-based lubricant, because of its long-lasting properties (Pure Romance's Pure Pleasure). The anus is made up of very delicate tissue and can tear easily, so you should always use plenty of silicone-based lubricant, and be prepared to reapply the lubricant as needed. A good rule here is that when you think you've used enough lubricant, use some more! When you're having fun with any kind of anal play, it's also important to keep in mind some basic hygienic practices, to keep you and your partner safe. You should use a latex or polyurethane condom with any toy that you'll be inserting into the rectum. This will prevent the transfer of bacteria from the anus to other parts of the body. For example, you and your partner might be having anal sex and then decide to stop, either because it's uncomfortable or because you want to move on to another type of sexual play. You might be considering going from anal sex to vaginal penetration. This is perfectly safe and okay to do, but you'll want to remove the condom used for anal sex before you begin vaginal sex. This will keep any bacteria from spreading to your vagina. With plenty of condoms and lubrication on hand, this kind of play can be both safe and comfortable!

Some people will find they do not enjoy anal sex, but others list it as their favorite type of sexual activity. After all, the anus is filled with nerve endings so it makes sense that it can be a rich source of pleasure for both the person penetrating and the person being penetrated. Like other kinds of sexual activities, some people will experience orgasm from anal intercourse, and others will not. It is normal for anal sex to be uncomfortable the first time you try it—just like vaginal intercourse—but it should *not* be painful. If you experience pain, take this as a sign from your body to stop. You can try again later during that same sexual experience. You can try again the next day, the next month, twenty years from now, or never again. Anal sex is a very personal decision and you should not be pressured into it. The better you and your partner are able to communicate your desires, the more likely it is you'll be able to take this step comfortably and without anxiety. On the other hand, deciding to experiment with anal play when you're ready and interested can make this one of the most exciting aspects to a couple's variety-filled sensual life.

ASK PATTY:
Unsure About Anal

Dear Patty,

My husband has expressed his desire to try anal sex. I have had one very bad experience with it and cannot seem to relax enough to even give in to the idea. But I know he really wants this and I want to make him happy. I have seen things that are supposed to help get your mind in the right place to get over your inhibitions. Do you recommend any of this stuff? And if so, what do you recommend?

Thanks.

Unsure about Anal

Dear Unsure about Anal,

Thanks for your question. Many people consider anal sex at some point during their life, and I applaud you for seeking out information before trying it a second time—since, as you guessed, there's definitely information you should know. Not every experience with anal intercourse is unpleasant; you may just need more information before you try it again.

Tearing can and does often happen, particularly when you're first trying to have anal sex, so you want to learn how to relax those muscles. Unlike the vagina, the rectum does not produce natural lubrication. Therefore, the general rule as far as a lubricant and anal sex goes is to use more than you think you could possibly want to use—and then still add more. The use of a silicone-based lubricant, such as Pleasure, will help prevent tearing and increase comfort.

Because of your apprehension with anal intercourse and your previous bad experience, I'd also like to suggest that you take this slowly by experimenting with insertion of your partner's finger prior to trying his penis. Again, use lots of lubricant, and maybe even a numbing cream. Your partner could put a condom over his finger—this would protect him from infection in case he had a cut on his finger; it would also protect you in the case that he had a blood-borne infection and a cut on his finger.

Even with all of the precautions listed above, it's important to emphasize that you need to feel comfortable with anal play. If you experience any pain, then you should back off and make sure you used the proper lubricant and let your body relax enough.

And remember, it's always preferable to use a condom when having anal sex to avoid transferring bacteria from the anus to your vagina. If you start having anal sex, and then decide to resume penile-vaginal intercourse, then you will want to remove the condom used for anal sex before your partner inserts his penis into your vagina. You want to make sure that bacteria from the anus do not get spread to your vagina. The same cleanliness rule applies if you are using a toy or fingers.

I think it's terrific that you and your partner have been able to talk openly about his interest in trying anal sex, and that you've kept an open mind about trying new things and seeking out information. I hope this is helpful for you in your decision. Good luck and have fun!

Truly,
Patty

A Calendar of Connections

One of the ways that a couple can move beyond missionary and infuse their relationship with excitement and energy is by deepening their connection. Intimacy is not only a sexual dimension in a relationship, it is also made up of a sense of fun, play, nonsexual touching, and showing each other you care. Consider this Calendar of Connections as your month-to-month guide to making sure you and your partner stay in touch—emotionally and physically.

January—Start Something New: A Journal

Use the arrival of a new calendar year to begin keeping a diary or journal, something many of us have done at least one time in our lives. Keeping a relationship journal is one way to express your feelings about your partner and your intimate relationship—feelings that change month to month, year to year. Try writing down those feelings along with your concerns, desires, and maybe even a fantasy. If you are having trouble with intimacy, noting the frequency of your sexual thoughts may reveal a pattern in your cycle of arousal, such as when you are feeling most aroused, how long, and what triggers it. You can use this for your own and your partner's benefit. Try copying a page from your journal and leaving it somewhere so your partner will find it. Reading about your thoughts and fantasies will open up a whole new form of communication.

February—Create a Simple Wish List

Reintroducing the simple pleasures and small gestures of romance into your relationship will help you both to continue to grow as a couple. On separate sheets of paper each of you should make a list of the small things your partner does regularly that make you feel loved. Put down everything you can think of—holding your hand in the car, kissing you at the end of the day, or getting your coffee in the morning. Then, add three small things you wish your partner would do more often or just once or twice. These could be things like bring home dinner, rub your feet, dance with you in the living room, read to you, or even bring you flowers. Now, exchange lists. Without discussing it, try to do one thing from your partner's list each day. It's the small things that matter in life, especially when you face difficult times in your relationship. Maybe you want to see him in a pair of sexy boxers, or suggest going to work out together. The point is to do things that show you care. Yes, buying a card or flowers is nice, but it's also typical. What about picking up a bag of Doritos if that's his favorite snack? Or doing some of the household chores without having to ask?

March—Do Something New Together

Take a cooking class, go ballroom dancing, attend a spin class or even a wine class together. Doing an activity as a couple can solidify your relationship in a new, exciting way. Why do you think *Dancing with the Stars* is so popular? What we are watching is a couple moving in sync. This is a metaphor for what you are trying to do: find your rhythm together.

Remember the feelings that came along with dating, when you were getting to know each other in so many different ways, including physically and sexually? The silliness and the laughing, sharing stories, learning about likes and dislikes, and finding out what turns each other on? Wouldn't you like to recapture that sense of excitement, and a little of the thrill of the unknown? So take some time to think about what the two of you might enjoy: if he likes to work with his hands, seek out a boat-building workshop. If you both like water, try sailing or scuba lessons. Activities take planning; they don't just happen—so give it some thought and you just might stumble upon a new passion the two of you can share for years to come.

April—Get Away!

Getting away for a night is a great way to restore the excitement in your relationship. Of course, taking a longer vacation together is ideal, but most of us can't afford the time and the expense, or we're reluctant to leave our kids for more than a night or two. But you don't have to go far to get the same effect of being away from everything. Stay at a local bed and breakfast you've always heard about, or visit a cabin nearby. Breaking the monotony of your normal routine can provide a renewed sense of closeness in your relationship. Intimacy is very important to couples, and if you and your partner have found that this aspect of your relationship has lost its spice, it's time to shake things up a bit. Choose someplace with a romantic atmosphere, preferably one with a cozy restaurant nearby. Begin with a wonderful candlelight dinner, then proceed to the room that you have reserved. Setting the mood with candles and dim lighting will help. Remember that intimacy is about more than just intercourse. Plan a nice relaxing bubble bath together and an evening of just lying in one another's arms. A night dedicated to just the two of you will go a long way toward rekindling your intimate relationship.

May—Offer a Springtime Massage

Giving your partner a massage when he (or she) is not feeling well or is worn out and tired can restore a feeling of closeness to your relationship. A massage can be a very sensual and intimate experience. Soft lighting, music, and a massage oil can help set the mood and create a comfortable environment for your partner to relax. Offering a massage lets your partner know that you recognize his need for a little extra attention. He (or she) will appreciate your thoughtfulness and this gesture will help improve your intimate relationship in the long run, both emotionally and physically.

June—Do a Mid-Year Review

If you've been keeping a relationship journal since January, take the time now to review it. Read back over your questions, your desires, your notes to yourself. Have you noticed any changes with your partner? Do you feel closer? Perhaps make a list of all that you are grateful for in your relationship. Next, write down aspects of your relationship you would like to change. How far apart are these two lists? What can you realistically expect to change and what are you able to accept, realizing that some things won't change. Healthy and happy relationships that last are often grounded in reality. Use this mid-year review to give yourself a reality check.

July—Take Care of Yourself

Summer is the best time to pay positive attention to your health. And as you know, the healthier you are, the more sexual you will feel. So now is the time to review your own and your partner's sexual health. Go back over the questions you asked yourself in Chapter 3 and ask yourself if you have noted any changes in your health that may be impacting your desire, arousal, or sexual responsiveness. One of the most crucial aspects about staying connected to your partner is feeling good about yourself. Focus on your positive features and limit your tendency to dwell on what you don't like about your appearance. Instead, try to boost your energy and your sense of well-being by taking good care of your health. Exercise. Eat right. Watch bad habits that sap your energy. Women should not forget the many other ways to enhance sexuality, including creating a relaxed, comfortable environment with soft music, lighting, candles, and food that encourages intimacy and sensuality.

August—Tap Into Your Senses

It's August and most of us are hot—inside and out. Take this steamy month at the end of summer as an opportunity to review how you and your partner get turned on. Science and sexuality have become believable bedfellows of late. More and more research and studies are showing just how our physiology and psychology impact and guide our sexual interests, libido, and responsiveness.

But one thing that science can't capture exactly is just what turns us on. For some people, it's a glimpse of an ankle in a red stiletto; for others, it's soft porn on the Internet or in the glossy pages of a magazine. Still others get aroused by the ripple of a wave, a warm, soft breeze across a naked shoulder, or a majestic view of the sunset as it sinks beyond the Pacific.

The more we can tap into what gets us hot and bothered, what physically turns us on, the more likely we will be able to become sexually fulfilled. Here are some questions to help you and your partner become more sensually aware:

1. Are you a visual person? Do you find yourself
   aroused by an image in print or video?

2. Are you an auditory person? Does a particular kind of music—with words or without—relax you and make your mind turn to things sexual?

3. Are you a tactile person? In order to get aroused, do you need to be caressed, kissed, or touched in a specific way?

4. Are you an oral person? Does a tender, moist kiss get you most excited? A nice glass of red wine? A sweet taste of dark chocolate?

5. Do you have a strong sense of smell? Does the scent of your lover turn you on? The waft of a cinnamon candle, or scent of your choice?

Usually, sexual arousal is triggered in part by one or more of our five senses. When we pay attention to our sensuality in this way, we can learn to fire up our sexuality and make it hot, hot, hot!

September—Schedule a Date Night

Okay, it might be back to school time for the kids, but it's also time to put your date night back on your schedule. Though you see each other daily and even go out to dinner every Friday night, setting up a date night outside of your usual schedule will enhance your relationship and bring special attention to each other. Treat each of these occasions as if they were first dates. Go all out getting yourself dressed up and take special care with your appearance. Prepare for your date night as if you were really trying to make a good first impression. Going out of your way to have at least one night of fun and romance a week will help add a little zing to your relationship. But even once a month is good—whatever works for you and your schedule—just make sure it happens. A simple night out can do wonders. And don't use the excuse of being afraid to leave your kids. I know one couple who was afraid to leave their kids with a babysitter, so they went to the lower level of their house and created a romantic space with a wine cellar as its focal point. They were finally able to enjoy this special area one night. They made a special dinner and had a wonderful time while one of the older kids in the neighborhood was upstairs watching their children. Set aside the time and find what works for you and your family. And remember, there is no one right thing to do or right time to do it.

October—Share Your Memories

Autumn is often a time people find themselves pondering favorite childhood memories. Sharing these memories and their meanings with each other can bring a couple closer. Have each of you take a piece of paper and record two or three of your most significant childhood memories. Examples may include favorite family events, rituals, holidays, or a time with a favorite family friend or relative. Next to each memory, record the most important element of the event. What was it about this event that was so meaningful to you? Record the main feeling that was associated with the memory. Then take turns sharing memories with your partner. Remind each other of your favorite moments together and why they mean so much. If you're married, look at your wedding album together. Or just talk through funny moments about the night you first met. Now, find a simple way to re-create the essence of that experience in your current life together. The goal is to allow yourself a few moments of fun and freedom, to honor a memorable and positive time in your life, and to share that experience with your partner so you feel closer and more connected.

November—Games People Play

As the weather begins to pull you inside, you might think about how you and your partner can play a game to spice up your relationship. Try reading the sexual position book (see Resources) or pick up a book of erotica.

You can also vary your lovemaking with a game, in which you number the various positions (front entry, rear entry, etc.) and then write down different positions on separate pieces of paper. Match the number with the position and off you go! This is an especially easy, fun game for couples who are not so verbal—the game-like approach helps take the heat off and smoothes out the tension of introducing something new.

Bedroom games allow couples to have fun and open lines of communication at the same time. Remember, strengthening and renewing your bonds of communication isn't all about heavy, serious talk. It can and should be light and fun, not to mention sexy and hot! Most important, games are a great way to relax, take the pressure off, and give yourself the freedom to explore.

Some couples also enjoy texting each other, suggesting what they want to do to each other or setting a time to meet—nothing is more sexy or creates more anticipation then opening a text message at work from your partner wanting you!

If you've discovered a secret fantasy or two that you're not quite sure how to share with your partner, you can write it down on paper and place it under his pillow, under the visor of his car, or put it in his pocket so he finds it when he goes for his keys.

The idea of adding this playful element into your sex life is to take the seriousness out and replace it with fun.

December—Laugh!

Laughter is sometimes the best medicine for whatever ails us, and a sense of humor is an absolute must for couples who want to stay in touch and in tune. Taking time away from your worries and responsibilities to laugh a little with your partner can do wonders for the two of you. Go to your local movie rental place and get your favorite comedy. If you are up for it—rent two! Make some popcorn and have your very own movie night! Dim the lights, relax on the couch together, and enjoy a night of laughing. You can't feel angry, upset, or sad at what is going on in your life if you are laughing—it is important to add laughter and fun back into your routine! You'll find that it will only improve your relationship. Never underestimate the value of spontaneity in a relationship. Too often, a relationship loses its sense of worth because it is overshadowed by the stresses of everyday life.

Some people jump to the conclusion that if one night or one encounter is not wild or passionate, then their sex life is over. It's unrealistic to think that your sexual or intimate relationship is always going to be passionate, and it's important to adjust your expectations so you don't put too much pressure on yourself, your partner, or your relationship. When you learn to celebrate the fun you have together and when you strengthen that deeper level of

Be Proactive

When you're single and interested in dating or meeting a partner, it's important to open your horizons and think outside the box. You've also got to be proactive and realistic. There *are* quality single people out there looking for relationships. They may not fit your ideal fantasy, but maybe it's time to set realistic standards and look for what really counts, like character and responsibility. On the other hand, if you're happy and content being on your own, savor this "me time" while you have it. Below are what I hope you will find inspiring tips on finding a new partner with whom to share your time, or some ideas to make your "me time" that much more enjoyable and satisfying.

♡ Look to the people you know—and tell them you'd really appreciate an introduction to a quality person, a serious date. Don't be shy. Your social network has resources for you to tap, but you've got to let your friends know what you're looking for and talk up your hopes.

♡ Check out the new-style bookstores or coffee shops and utilize them for socializing. Upscale grocery stores also have great reputations as scenes for meeting new people. Some even have singles nights! Check your local paper.

♡ Get involved in local politics, join an exercise center, or volunteer at your local hospital. Whether looking for a Friday night date or some platonic comraderie, the more you do, the more people you'll meet.

♡ Take a night class in computer programming, financial planning, or a carpentry course. You never know who you'll meet who shares that interest. And if you're not looking to meet someone, you will definitely exercise your brain—always a good thing!

♡ Find out what activities your community center, church, or synagogue provides for single members to get together. These venues often draw like-minded people, who share your values.

♡ Take out a personal ad, or answer one. Email lets you keep your anonymity until you're ready to jump in. (When you're ready to meet in person, it's wise to do so in public places, until you feel confident that the person you've met is trustworthy.)

♡ Use a dating service. Of course, Match.com, eHarmony, and It's Just Lunch are some of the more popular choices across the country. But don't overlook the smaller, boutique dating services that might be more locally based.

♡ Buy an irresistible dog or a quirky, sexy car. If a car is out of the question, how about a stylish new outfit?

communication, you give your relationship the tools and the foundation for getting through those periods when it's not hot and heavy.

It's so important to appreciate what you have now in your relationship, while always remembering that every relationship changes. And through periods of change, it becomes more important than ever to focus on the positive. Sure, you can focus on what things used to be like—sometimes it's good to reminisce—but don't get stuck on comparisons with how things used to be. And the same is true of comparing yourselves to other couples or wishing for something different or new. It's an old cliché but it's true: The grass is not always greener on other side; it just needs more mowing.

Trust yourself, listen to yourself. You will know in your gut what is right—or wrong—for you. We often take more time selecting the right cantaloupe then we do selecting what is right in our relationship.

When it comes to a relationship, if it's worth having, it's worth working for. And just like it's not realistic to count on instant wealth by winning the lottery or landing an inheritance, when it comes to your intimate relationship, you need to continually work to know your body, your partner's, and where you two meet.

Acknowledgments

WRITING MY FIRST book was quite an extraordinary experience and I want to thank all of the people who helped make this book possible. First, I would like to thank my agents, Lisa Queen and Eleanor Jackson, for their wise advice, warm encouragement, and faithful support throughout this process. I am particularly grateful for my collaborator, Billie Fitzpatrick, who diligently and creatively took my voice and all of my experience and crafted it onto the page. I would also like to extend my great appreciation to my publishing team at Atria, Judith Curr, Gary Urda, Christine Duplessis, Christine Saunders, and most especially my inspiring, learned editor Greer Hendricks, and the ever-helpful Sarah Walsh.

And of course, I would also like to thank my wonderful team at Pure Romance, especially Kim Sheridan and Erin Lapham, M.P.H., whose editorial and research involvement were invaluable. I am particularly grateful for all of the Pure Romance Consultants who have gone above and beyond the role of saleswomen. They are truly committed to helping women in regard to their sexual health and are continuously striving to learn more and provide more information to this end.

In addition, I have always said that I would not have been able to touch so many women's lives without the support and efforts of the researchers, experts, and the medical community who have rallied behind Pure Romance—most specifically, Dr. Michael Reece and Dr. Debby Herbenick, The Center for Sexual Health Promotion and Indiana University, Dr. Rachel Pauls, Dr. Mickey Karram, Dr. William Jamieson, the National Vulvodynia Association, The American Association of Sexuality Educators, Counselors and Therapists, the Wellness Community of Greater Cincinnati and Northern Kentucky, the Susan G. Komen Foundation Cincinnati Affiliate, the Young Survival Coalition, and Living Beyond Breast Cancer.

A special thanks to Susan Colvin and Jackie White, Paul and Barbara Mandel, and Loren and Moe Levy who have all worked closely with Pure Romance to ensure that every product we carry always lives up to our highest expectations.

Last, but certainly not least, I want to thank my family—especially my son, Chris, for helping me to realize my goals, follow my passion, and see the bigger picture when it came to my business; my children, Nick, Matt, and Lauren for making my passion their own; and my parents, for teaching me the importance of a strong work ethic and staying focused no matter what obstacles were to come my way.

Resources

Books

Allison, Sadie. *Tickle Your Fancy: A Woman's Guide to Sexual Self Pleasure.* San Francisco: Tickle Kitty Press, 2001.

Allison, Sadie. *Tickle His Pickle: Your Hands-On Guide to Penis Pleasuring.* San Francisco: Tickle Kitty Press, 2004.

Alterowitz, Ralph, and Barbara Alterowitz. *Intimacy with Impotence: The Couple's Guide to Better Sex after Prostate Disease.* Massachusetts: Da Capo Lifelong Books, 2004.

The Boston Women's Health Book Collective. *Our Bodies, Ourselves.* New York: Simon & Schuster, 2005.

The Boston Women's Health Book Collective and Vivian Pinn. *Our Bodies, Ourselves: Menopause.* New York: Simon & Schuster, 2006.

Ferrer, Charley. *The W.I.S.E. Journal for the Sensual Woman.* Seattle: Hara Publishing, 2001.

Fincannon, Joy, RN, MS, and Katherine Bruss, PsyD. *Couples*

Confronting Cancer: Keeping Your Relationship Strong. American Cancer Society, 2003.

Glazer, Howard I., Ph.D., and Gae Rodke, M.D., FACOG. *The Vulvodynia Survival Guide: How to Overcome Painful Vaginal Symptoms and Enjoy an Active Lifestyle.* Oakland, CA: New Harbinger Publications, Inc., 2002.

Heiman, Julia, R., Ph.D., and Joseph Lopiccolo, Ph.D. *Becoming Orgasmic: A Sexual and Personal Growth Program for Women.* New York: Prentice Hall Press, 1988.

Kaufmann, Miriam, M.D., Corey Silverberg, and Fran Odette. *The Ultimate Guide to Sex and Disability.* San Francisco: Cleis Press, 2003.

Link, John, M.D. *The Breast Cancer Survivor Manual: A Step-by-Step Guide for the Woman with Newly Diagnosed Breast Cancer, 4th Edition.* New York: Henry Holt and Company, 2007.

Margot, Sandra, Deborah Herman, and Tonianne Robino. *The Pregnant Couple's Guide to Sex, Romance, and Intimacy: Everything you Need to Know to Preserve your Relationship During and After Pregnancy.* New York: Citadel, 2002.

National Women's Health Resource Center. *Fast Facts: Understanding Vaginal Pain and Vulvodynia.* National Women's Health Resource Center, 2005.

Pertot, Sandra, Ph.D. *Perfectly Normal: Living and Loving with Low Libido.* Emmaus, PA: Rodale, Inc., 2005.

Roszler, Janis, and Donna Rice. *Sex and Diabetes.* American Diabetes Association, 2007.

Shulman, Neil, M.D., and Edmund Kim, M.D., OB/GYN. *Healthy Transitions: A Woman's Guide to Perimenopause, Menopause, and Beyond.* New York: Prometheus Books, 2004.

Snellen, Martien. *Sex and Intimacy after Childbirth*. Australia: Text Publishing, 2005.

Stewart, Elizabeth, M.D., and Paula Spencer. *The V Book: A Doctor's Guide to Complete Vulvovaginal Health*. New York: Bantam Books, 2002.

Stewart, Jessica. *The Complete Guide to Sexual Positions*, 4th Edition. Los Angeles: Pacific Media, 2007.

Wincze, John, and Michael Carey. *Sexual Dysfunction: A Guide for Assessment and Treatment*, 2nd Edition. New York: Guilford Press, 2001.

WEBSITES

American Association of Marriage and Family Therapy: www.aamft.org

The American Association of Sexuality Educators, Counselors and Therapists: www.aasect.org

American Cancer Society: www.cancer.org

American Menopause Foundation: www.americanmenopause.org

Association of Reproductive Health Professionals, Menopause Resource Center: www.arhp.org

The Centers for Disease Control and Prevention: www.cdc.gov

Female Sexual Dysfunction Online: www.femalesexualdysfunctiononline.org

National Institute on Aging: www.nia.nih.gov

National Vulvodynia Association: www.nva.org

National Women's Health Network: www.nwhn.org

The National Women's Health Information Center: www.4women.gov

The North American Menopause Society: www.menopause.org

Planned Parenthood Federation of America: www.plannedparent hood.org

Rape, Abuse, and Incest National Network (RAINN): www .rainn.org

The Sexual Assault Resource Agency: www.sexualassaultresources .org

The Susan G. Komen Breast Cancer Foundation: www.komen .org

The Women's Sexual Health Foundation: www.twshf.org

The Young Survival Coalition: www.youngsurvival.org

Medications That Can Impact Libido and Arousal in Women

Medications that may cause disorders of desire	Medications that may cause disorders of arousal
PSYCHOACTIVE MEDICATIONS	— Anticholinergics
— Antipsychotics	— Antihistamines
— Barbiturates	— Antihypertensives
— Benzodiazepines	PSYCHOACTIVE MEDICATIONS
— Lithium	— Benzodiazepines
— Selective serotonin reuptake inhibitors	— Selective serotonin reuptake inhibitors
— (SSRIs)	— Monoamine oxidase inhibitors
— Tricyclic antidepressants	— Tricyclic antidepressants

Cardiovascular and antihypertensive medications	Medications that may cause orgasmic disorders
— Antilipid medications — Beta blockers — Clonidine — Digoxin — Spironolactone	— Amphetamines and related anorexic drugs — Antipsychotics — Benzodiazepines — Mehyldopa — Narcotics — Selective serotonin reuptake inhibitors — Trazodone — Tricyclic antidepressants*
Hormonal preparations	
— Danazol — Gn-RH agonists — Oral contraceptives	
Other	*Also associated with painful orgasm Adapted from: "Drugs that cause sexual dysfunction: an update." *Med Lett Drugs Ther* 1992; 34:73-78.
— Histamine H2-receptor blockers and promotility agents — Indomethacin — Ketoconazole — Phenytoin sodium	

BOOKS FOR PLEASURE

Barbach, Lonnie. *For Each Other: Sharing Sexual Intimacy.* New York: Anchor, 1982.

Blue, Violet, ed. *Best Women' Erotica, 2008.* San Francisco: Cleis, 2008.

Blue, Violet, ed. *The Ultimate Guide to Adult Videos: How to Watch*

Adult Videos and Make Your Sex Life Sizzle. San Francisco: Cleis, 2002.

Cohen, Angela, and Sarah Gardner Fox. *The Wise Woman's Guide to Erotic Videos: 300 Sexy Videos for Every Woman—and Her Lover.* New York: Broadway, 1997.

Bibliography

A note about the Bibliography: the references listed here comprise those sources referred to or consulted during the writing of this book.

Booth, Rebecca, M.D. *The Venus Week.* Cambridge, MA: Da Capo, 2008.

Both, S., Spiering, M., Everaerd, W., Laan, E. (2004). "Sexual behavior and responsiveness to sexual stimuli following laboratory-induced sexual arousal." *Journal of Sex Research*, 41(3):242–58.

Dodson, Betty. *Sex for One.* New York: Three Rivers Press, 1996.

Holstein, Lana, M.D. *How to Have Magnificent Sex.* New York: Crown, 2001.

Ladas Kahn, Alice, Beverly Whipple, and John Perry. *The G-Spot: And Other Recent Discoveries about Human Sexuality.* New York: Dell, 1982.

Lindberg, Marrena, *The Orgasmic Diet.* New York: Three Rivers Press, 2007.

Paget, Lou. *The Big O.* New York: Gotham, 2006.

Web Studies

www.webmd.com/sex-relationships/guide/20061101/sex-better-
     than-money-for-happiness
www.twshf.org

Printed in the United States
By Bookmasters